Towards a Social Science of Drugs in Sport

The debate around the role of drugs in sport is vibrant. There is a wealth of evidence from the hard end of science, telling us how drugs work, how drug testing works, and how many athletes have fallen foul of the system. The evidence from social science is still building momentum. For example, what makes an athlete use a performance enhancing substance? "To win" simply fails to explain the drug use behaviour we see among athletes.

This book provides a foundation for anyone trying to understand the drugs in sport problem beyond the hard science by looking at the "people factor" from different perspectives. After building a case for the social science of drugs in sport, it is examined from the ethical, sociological, economic, legal and psychological points of view. The book concludes with a definitive statement about what researchers, policy makers, sports administrators, athletes and fans can do to achieve a social science of drugs in sport that puts people firmly in the centre of the debate.

This book was previously published as a special issue of *Sport in Society.*

Jason Mazanov is a Senior Lecturer at the UNSW Canberra Campus. Dr Mazanov started his career as a Health Psychologist before moving into the social science of drugs in sport. This move has seen Dr Mazanov develop expertise as a sports policy and management researcher.

Towards a Social Science of Drugs in Sport

Edited by
Jason Mazanov

Routledge
Taylor & Francis Group
LONDON AND NEW YORK

First published 2012
by Routledge
2 Park Square, Milton Park, Abingdon, Oxon, OX14 4RN

Simultaneously published in the USA and Canada
by Routledge
605 Third Avenue, New York, NY 10017

Routledge is an imprint of the Taylor & Francis Group, an informa business

First issued in paperback 2013

This book is a reproduction of *Sport in Society*, vol. 12, issue 3. The Publisher requests to those authors who may be citing this book to state, also, the bibliographical details of the special issue on which the book was based.

British Library Cataloguing in Publication Data
A catalogue record for this book is available from the British Library

ISBN13: 978-0-415-85314-9 (pbk)
ISBN13: 978-0-415-68586-3 (hbk)

Typeset in Times New Roman
by Taylor & Francis Books

Disclaimer
The publisher would like to make readers aware that the chapters in this book are referred to as articles as they had been in the special issue. The publisher accepts responsibility for any inconsistencies that may have arisen in the course of preparing this volume for print.

Contents

SPORT IN THE GLOBAL SOCIETY –
CONTEMPORARY PERSPECTIVES

Series Editor: Boria Majumdar

TOWARDS A SOCIAL SCIENCE OF DRUGS IN SPORT

Sport in the Global Society – Contemporary Perspectives

Series Editor: Boria Majumdar

The social, cultural (including media) and political study of sport is an expanding area of scholarship and related research. While this area has been well served by the *Sport in the Global Society* series, the surge in quality scholarship over the last few years has necessitated the creation of *Sport in the Global Society: Contemporary Perspectives.* The series will publish the work of leading scholars in fields as diverse as sociology, cultural studies, media studies, gender studies, cultural geography and history, political science and political economy. If the social and cultural study of sport is to receive the scholarly attention and readership it warrants, a cross-disciplinary series dedicated to taking sport beyond the narrow confines of physical education and sport science academic domains is necessary. *Sport in the Global Society: Contemporary Perspectives* will answer this need.

Titles in the Series

Australian Sport
Antipodean Waves of Change
Edited by Kristine Toohey and Tracy Taylor

Australia's Asian Sporting Context
1920s and 1930s
Edited by Sean Brawley and Nick Guoth

'Critical Support' for Sport
Bruce Kidd

Disability in the Global Sport Arena
A Sporting Chance
Edited by Jill M. Clair

Diversity and Division – Race, Ethnicity and Sport in Australia
Christopher J. Hallinan

Documenting the Beijing Olympics
Edited by D. P. Martinez

Football in Brazil
Edited by Martin Curi

Football Supporters and the Commercialisation of Football
Comparative Responses across Europe
Edited by Peter Kennedy and David Kennedy

Football's Relationship with Art: The Beautiful Game?
John E. Hughson

Forty Years of Sport and Social Change, 1968-2008
"To Remember is to Resist"
Edited by Russell Field and Bruce Kidd

Global Perspectives on Football in Africa
Visualising the Game
Edited by Susann Baller, Giorgio Miescher and Raffaele Poli

Global Sport Business
Community Impacts of Commercial Sport
Edited by Hans Westerbeek

Governance, Citizenship and the New European Football Championships
The European Spectacle
Edited by Wolfram Manzenreiter and Georg Spitaler

Indigenous People, Race Relations and Australian Sport
Edited by Christopher J. Hallinan and Barry Judd

Perspectives on Sport and Music
Perfect Pitch
Edited by Anthony Bateman

Reviewing UK Football Cultures
Continuing with Gender Analyses
Edited by Jayne Caudwell

Soccer in the Middle East
Edited by Issam Khalidi and Alon Raab

South Africa and the Global Game
Football, Apartheid and Beyond
Edited by Peter Alegi and Chris Bolsmann

Sport – Race, Ethnicity and Identity
Building Global Understanding
Edited by Daryl Adair

Sport and the Community
Edited by Allan Edwards and David Hassan

Sport, Culture and Identity in the State of Israel
Edited by Yair Galily and Amir Ben-Porat

Sport in Australian National Identity
Kicking Goals
Tony Ward

Sport in the City
Cultural Connections
Edited by Michael Sam and John E. Hughson

The Changing Face of Cricket
From Imperial to Global Game
Edited by Dominic Malcolm, Jon Gemmell and Nalin Mehta

The Consumption and Representation of Lifestyle Sports
Edited by Belinda Wheaton

The Containment of Soccer in Australia
Fencing Off the World Game
Edited by Christopher J. Hallinan and John E. Hughson

The Flame Relay and the Olympic Movement
John J. MacAloon

The History of Motor Sport
A Case Study Analysis
Edited by David Hassan

The Making of Sporting Cultures
John E. Hughson

The Olympic Movement and the Sport of Peacekeeping
Edited by Ramón Spaaij and Cindy Burleson

The Politics of Sport
Community, Mobility, Identity
Edited by Paul Gilchrist and Russell Holden

The Politics of Sport in South Asia
Edited by Subhas Ranjan Chakraborty, Shantanu Chakrabarti and Kingshuk Chatterjee

The Social Impact of Sport
Edited by Ramón Spaaij

Towards a Social Science of Drugs in Sport
Edited by Jason Mazanov

Who Owns Football?
The Governance and Management of the Club Game Worldwide
Edited by David Hassan and Sean Hamil

Why Minorities Play or Don't Play Soccer
A Global Exploration
Edited by Kausik Bandyopadhyay

Developing an agenda for social science research into drugs in sport

Jason Mazanov

School of Business, UNSW@ADFA, Canberra, Australia

This article provides a short introduction and overview to a collection of essays designed to provide a starting point in the form of a research agenda towards developing a social science of drugs in sport. It firstly addresses the paucity of social science research on the issues and then summarizes the approach taken to developing a research agenda to guide social science research into drugs in sport. This is done through describing the conceptual relationship between five pairs of essays comprising of the argument for a social science of drugs in sport (historical and overview of the development of the research agenda), developing policy (sport philosophy and sociology), implementing policy (economics and law), individual response to policy (health and educational psychology), and the research agenda (discipline specific and cosmopolitan).

There has been a massive amount of research into drugs in sport and anti-doping initiatives. A survey of the research literature demonstrates a formidable amount of medical and physical science research aimed at identifying athletes who seek advantage through banned performance-enhancing substances or methods. This represents what might be termed 'detection-based deterrence', or the idea that the prospect of getting caught using a prohibited substance will be enough to stop an athlete from using. While detection-based deterrence has had some success, attention is now turning to whether social science can inform 'prevention-based deterrence', or stopping an athlete from wanting to use prohibited substances or methods.[1]

When a survey of research literature is taken across the social sciences in relation to prevention-based deterrence it reveals two important things. The first is that there is surprisingly little research, and the second is that what exists is difficult to find.[2] In terms of what exists, there are a few unconnected studies from economics, psychology and sociology.[3] Thus, at the start of the twenty-first century there is surprisingly little in the way of systematic research by social scientists into performance-enhancing drug or method use by athletes.

Filling this gap in an organized way means working towards a social science of drugs in sport to answer some basic questions, such as 'Why do athletes take drugs?' and 'Why do we have drugs in sport in the first place?'[4] That is, developing a research agenda to guide the development of a social science of drugs in sport.

Development of the agenda reported in this collection was construed with two very specific aims in mind. The first was to provide an insight into how social science views drugs in sport. The second was to stimulate social science research into drugs in sport as a starting point to ask theoretically or empirically relevant questions, or provide points of contention with which to agree or disagree. Developing the agenda brought together a team of social scientists from economics, education, law, psychology, sociology and sports philosophy to outline some directions for future research from their discipline.

Structure of the agenda

Five pairs of essays make up the agenda. The first pair of essays is aimed at providing readers with grounding in the context of drugs in sport research. The first essay (Mazanov and McDermott) argues the case for developing a social science of drugs in sport using the historical evolution of the anti-doping policy. The purpose of the second essay (Mazanov) is to give readers some insight into what the contributors to the collection thought about and reflected upon when preparing their contributions. Specifically, it summarizes two workshops held to define what social science needs to do to best respond to the drugs in sport issue.

The second pair looks to explore the ideology underpinning drugs in sport research with sports philosophy and sociology. Anti-doping is the dominant ideology governing drugs in sport, presuming the role of drugs in sport is malignant and should be excised. While dominant, anti-doping is just one of many potential ideologies to guide the response to drugs in sport. Philosophy and sociology ask critical questions about where such ideologies come from and whether they are worth pursuing relative to other models, exploring the existing model as only one of several possible realities. The approach taken by the essays on sport philosophy (Hemphill) and sociology (Connor) are to critically evaluate the arguments used to support the anti-doping stance. The evaluation of these arguments leads to an exploration of ideas of what sport means to individuals and to societies in general. These arguments lead to questions about what humans want for sport, and whether drugs have a role to play.

Where the essays on philosophy and sociology explored ideologies that lead to particular policies about drugs in sport, the third pair of essays take the policies as somewhat more fixed and explores what they might mean in practice. This gives rise to a consideration of both the intended and unintended consequences of such policies that might emerge. By using the rational model as one against which to speculate about reality, Sharpe's application of economic theory to drugs in sport issues provides a method for assessing whether the operationalization of different ideologies and their policies leads to the expected outcomes. Once a policy has been decided upon, the law provides a wealth of experience in designing systems that define the rules and the authority to implement those rules (Amos and Fridman). This adds another layer of sophistication to exploring the intended and unintended consequences associated with the policy implementation of various ideologies.

The fourth pair of essays looks to how individuals respond within established ideological or policy systems, using the lens of psychology. Two sub-disciplines of psychology are considered here, health (Quirk) and educational (Hanson). Health psychology takes an interest in volitional behaviour that can influence the integrity of human functioning, such as suppression of immune function from overtraining, behaviours that increase the risk of disease, or the deliberate use of drugs known to be detrimental to longevity. Educational psychology is central to a discussion of drugs in sport as one of the foundations underpinning anti-doping activity, specifically its role in developing interventions that help athletes make decisions about their drug use behaviour. The educational psychologist might look at the drugs in sport issue as one focused on ensuring athletes draw on the information available to them at the critical decision point of use or abstinence.

The final pair of essays concludes the development of the research agenda by articulating a set of research questions that cuts across discipline boundaries (cosmopolitan research), and then defines the agenda. The aim of the cosmopolitan research agenda (Mazanov) is to inspire collaboration between disciplines towards cosmopolitan, rather than multidisciplinary, work.

Cosmopolitan work in this context is meant to encourage research that uses relevant ideas from a discipline because it helps explain some aspect of the drugs in sport phenomenon. The final essay in the collection (Mazanov) is intended as a stand alone statement to stimulate debate through robust and constructive examination of which ideas have merit and which need to be consigned to the dustbin of mediocrity. If the agenda can inspire researchers, policy makers or commentators to further the social science of drugs in sport, then it has achieved its purpose.

Acknowledgements

This work was funded by the Australian Government through the Anti-Doping Research Program, whose management of the project has been integral to its success. As with any such effort, many people make up the eventual success of the project. The project was given crucial momentum at its conception by Dr Anthony Millgate, Professor Stephen Mugford and Professor Peter Hall. Important contributions over the life of the project were made by Associate Professor Tim Rolfe, Dr Eugene Aidman, Mr Ken Norris, Mrs Alannah Kazlauskas and Mr Trevor O'Donnell. Professor Brian Stoddart made a significant contribution to the project with sound, measured advice. As the convenor of the project, my personal thanks go to the contributors to this collection who did much more than write, and to my family who shared the ride.

Notes

1. BMA, *Drugs in Sport.*
2. This is reinforced by the review of social psychological investigation of anti-doping by Backhouse *et al.*, *Attitudes, Behaviours, Knowledge and Education.*
3. These papers include Berentsen and Lengwiler, 'Fraudulent Accounting and other Doping Games'; Anshel, 'Causes for Drug Use in Sport'; Donovan *et al.*, 'A Conceptual Framework for Achieving Performance Enhancing Drug Compliance in Sport'; Mazanov *et al.*, 'Towards an Empirical Model of Performance Enhancing Supplement Use'; Strelan and Boeckmann, 'A New Model for Understanding Performance-enhancing Drug Use by Elite Athletes', and 'Why Drug Testing in Elite Sport does not Work'; Coakley, *Sports in Society*; and Waddington, *Sport, Health and Drugs.*
4. Answering either question with 'to win' is unlikely to be helpful when looking to develop, design or guide interventions.

References

Anshel, M.H. 'Causes for Drug Use in Sport: A Survey of Intercollegiate Athletes'. *Journal of Sport Behaviour* 14 (1991): 283–307.

Backhouse, S., J. McKenna, S. Robinson, and A. Atkin. *Attitudes, Behaviours, Knowledge and Education – Drugs in Sport: Past, Present and Future*. Montreal: World Anti-Doping Agency, 2007.

Berensten, A., and Y. Lengwiler. 'Fraudulent Accounting and other Doping Games'. *Journal of Institutional and Theoretical Economics* 160, no. 3 (2004): 402–15.

BMA. *Drugs in Sport: The Pressure to Perform.* London: BMJ Publishing Group, 2002.

Coakley, J. *Sports in Society: Issues and Controversies.* Sydney: McGraw-Hill, 2007.

Donovan, R.J., G. Egger, V. Kapernick, and J. Mendoza. 'A Conceptual Framework for Achieving Performance Enhancing Drug Compliance in Sport'. *Sports Medicine* 32, no. 4 (2002): 269–84.

Mazanov, J., A. Petroczi, J. Bingham, and A. Holloway. 'Towards an Empirical Model of Performance Enhancing Supplement Use: A Pilot Study among High Performance UK Athletes'. *Journal of Science and Medicine in Sport* 11, no. 2 (2008): 185–90.

Strelan, P., and R.J. Boeckmann. 'A New Model for Understanding Performance-enhancing Drug Use by Elite Athletes'. *Journal of Applied Sport Psychology* 15 (2003): 176–83.

Strelan, P., and R.J. Boeckmann. 'Why Drug Testing in Elite Sport does not Work: Perceptual Deterrence Theory and the Role of Personal Moral Beliefs'. *Journal of Applied Social Psychology* 36 (2006): 2909–34.

Waddington, I. *Sport, Health and Drugs: A Critical Sociological Perspective*. London: E & FN Spon, 2000.

The case for a social science of drugs in sport

Jason Mazanov[a] and Vanessa McDermott[b]

[a]*School of Business, UNSW@ADFA, Canberra, Australia;* [b]*Department of Sociology, Australian National University, Canberra, Australia*

Social science began to take a prominent role in drugs in sport research in the early twenty-first century. This development has its roots in the history of drugs in sport, from the ancient Olympics through to the twentieth century, where the question of 'could' drugs enhance sporting performance, answered affirmatively, was replaced with whether they 'should'. The history of drug testing reveals that 'should' may have been asked too late, with the advent of potentially undetectable performance enhancements rendering testing ineffective as a deterrence method. In an effort to find alternative models to deter the use of drugs in sport, the focus has shifted from 'detection-based deterrence' to 'prevention-based deterrence'. Many of the questions underpinning prevention-based deterrence have the character of those asked by social science. Exploration of this character demonstrates social science offers an appropriate range of philosophical and methodological tools to explore prevention-based deterrence of drugs in sport.

An observer of drugs in sport issues in Germany through the 1930s[1] claimed it would be futile to discuss the issue on 'any but a medical basis'. Some 70 years later there is mounting evidence[2] other approaches may hold promise in contributing to discussion on drugs in sport, one such approach being that offered by social science. The case for social science is founded upon an examination of the evolution of anti-doping policies and the exploration of alternatives to this policy. Understanding the evolution of anti-doping policies towards these alternatives means developing the history of drugs in sport (from ancient to modern times) as background.

A brief history of drugs in sport

To establish a working knowledge for a discussion of drugs in sport, it is useful to have some idea of how the use of drugs in sport has evolved over time. The historical overview commences with identifying why drugs in sport issues are commonly referred to as 'anti-doping'. The first step in the process of developing the story of drugs in sport is to define 'doping' in both an historical and contemporary sense.[3]

What is doping?

While there were a number of doping scandals in the last 30 or 40 years of the twentieth century it would be incorrect to assume that doping emerged at this time.[4] The word doping is believed to have originated from an eighteenth-century drink known as '*dop*', which was a type of South African brandy consisting of walnut extract, xanthines and alcohol. This drink was used to improve endurance in ceremonial dances. The sporting connection to doping can be traced to the use of *dop* in the nineteenth century to describe a narcotic potion given to racehorses. By the turn of the twentieth century, doping described the methods and substances given to racehorses to *reduce* their chance of winning and influence the outcome of bets. The term 'doping' grew to include the use of substances that alter sporting competitors' performance.

In contemporary terms, doping refers to the misuse of drugs and includes methods designed to improve sporting performance or to manipulate doping tests. The International Olympic Committee (IOC) defines doping as:

1. The use of an expedient (substance or method) which is potentially harmful to the athlete's health and/or capable of enhancing their performance;
2. The presence in the athlete's body of a prohibited substance or evidence of the use thereof or evidence of the use of a prohibited method.[5]

However, the use of substances to improve sporting performances is by no means a twentieth-century phenomenon.

An historical view of drug use in sport

In the sixth century, dried figs were an essential part of an athlete's diet until superseded by meat which was believed to provide the strength of ten.[6] Stimulants such as herbal mixtures, wild mushrooms and plant seeds were also used.[7] These practices were not considered cheating and there are no recorded doping scandals at the ancient Olympics.[8] Warriors such as the Berserkers of Norse mythology, Roman gladiators and medieval knights were often described using magic potions or other substances for their stimulating effects and to overcome injury.

At the turn of the twentieth century, a range of drugs and other substances were commonly used in sport.[9] For example, Dutch canal swimmers used ether-soaked sugar cubes and distance runners, sprinters and cyclists are recorded to have used some, or any, combination of caffeine, alcohol, nitroglycerine, digitalis, cocaine, strychnine, ether, opium or heroin.[10] Although a widespread and accepted practice, these substances also carried significant risks. In 1896, it is alleged that cyclist Arthur Linton died after being given strychnine by his coach.[11] At the 1904 Olympic Marathon British athlete Thomas Hicks came close to death after using a mixture of strychnine and brandy.

Through the late nineteenth century, attention to doping was limited to a medical interest in the combined effect of sporting exertion and substances on human physiology. In 1894, sports physician Philippe Tissié studied the effects of stimulants on the performance of a long distance cyclist. Tissié's interest was entirely medical and based on the danger that athletes could die of athletic stress. While anti-doping policies did emerge at the turn of the nineteenth century, this took place in horseracing and was driven by the need to protect gamblers interests. Doping was considered unfair to gamblers who had no way of knowing which horses were doped and was not concerned with the ethics of athletes' doping practices.

The history of anti-doping strategies

In 1903 the English Jockey Club prohibited doping and in 1910 a test was developed to detect the most common drugs. In 1928, the Amateur Athletic Foundation was the first human sporting organization to ban 'stimulating substances'.[12] However, there were no comprehensive anti-doping mechanisms in place in sport. While some governments restricted the availability of opium and cocaine to prescription only, other drugs such as laudanum remained available over the counter. Interest in doping and performance enhancing substances and methods (PESM) during the period from the turn of the twentieth century to 1960 can best be summed up by the practical question '*Could we?*' and was generally unconcerned with the moral question of '*Should we?*'

Could we? Doping from the early 1900s to 1960

Prior to the 1930s there was little objection to doping despite the fact that athletes were using a number of drugs long before this time. Part of the explanation for this is related to the changing nature of sport in the twentieth century. At the end of the nineteenth century elite athletes were a 'curiosity not a charismatic figure at the centre of huge commercial enterprises'.[13] As Hoberman notes,[14] this changed in the twentieth century as modern sports became a branch of the entertainment industry. For example, a 1939 paper entitled 'Doping' stated:

> There can be no doubt that stimulants are today widely used by athletes participating in competitions; the record-breaking craze and desire to satisfy an exacting public play a more and more prominent role, and take higher rank than the health of the competitors itself.[15]

The evolution of sport gained momentum following the Second World War as prize money increased. Consequently, rather than an emphasis on participation, the rewards associated with winning became a primary consideration. At the same time as sport became more commercialized, medical advances also influenced doping in sport.

It is unsurprising that athletes took advantage of advances in medical technology given the combination of an increasing acceptance of doping and an upward trend in monetary rewards. The 1930s saw the development of amphetamine-like stimulants which, although initially used by combat soldiers, became the drug of choice for athletes in the post-war years (1940s and 1950s). Just as some earlier athletes had died from PESM use, a number of deaths in the 1940s and 1950s continued to highlight the dangers of doping. For example, in September 1949 a racing cyclist died of amphetamine poisoning in Italy.

Nevertheless, sport governing bodies (SGBs) did little to address the issue. In the case of the IOC, a permissive stance was taken despite evidence of doping at the 1952 and 1956 Olympic Games. For example, at the 1952 Oslo Winter Olympics broken ampoules and injection syringes were found in speed skaters' locker rooms with several skaters requiring medical attention.[16] At the 1956 Melbourne Olympics similar evidence of doping was found in cyclists' locker rooms.[17] By the end of the 1950s, it was clear that the answer to '*Could we?*' was a resounding yes. However, following several highly public deaths in the 1960s, the moral question of '*Should we?*' came to the forefront of the doping issue.

Should we? Doping in the 1960s to 1980s

The first high profile sporting death was cyclist Knud Jensen who died at the 1960 Rome Olympics. The official cause of death was sunstroke; however, the autopsy revealed evidence of amphetamines. In addition, two of Jensen's teammates were taken to hospital in a toxic condition. Jensen was not the only athlete whose death was linked to PESM. In the same year, track athlete Dick Howard died after using 'pep pills'. However, there were no anti-doping rules at the 1960 Olympics and the IOC did not form a Medical Committee to investigate doping until 1962. While the IOC did pass a resolution condemning doping, little action followed and the Medical Committee did not produce a report for another three years.[18]

Admittedly, some of this delay can be attributed to the lack of organizational and management resources in the IOC at that time. However, a primary contributing factor was that doping was seen as a problem associated with professional sport. Amateur sport was idealized as important for the 'betterment of mankind' while professional sport was seen as a degraded form of sport.[19]

In the late 1950s and into the 1960s SGBs and governments were slow to respond to doping. In 1959 the Union Cycliste Internationale (UCI) was the first international SGB to introduce drug testing and in the 1960s other international SGBs, including the International Amateur Athletics Federation (IAAF),[20] developed anti-doping policies. The Council of Europe tabled a resolution against the use of doping substances in sport in 1960, and in 1963 developed a list of banned substances and a definition of doping.[21] Also in 1963, France introduced the first anti-doping legislation followed by Belgium in 1965. However, many SGBs refused to accept that doping was a problem and, where it was acknowledged, were convinced that the problem would soon be controlled by drug testing.

Throughout the 1960s, doping continued and the efforts of SGBs seemed lacking in purpose. For example, although the IAAF announced random spot checks in 1966, a medical committee was not formed until 1972. In football (soccer), random testing did not take place until the 1966 World Cup. The slow response to doping at this time was not due to a lack of technology, as the ability to detect some substances had been available since about 1910, with most commonly available substances detectable by about 1960. As the late Manfred Donike, drug testing pioneer, pointed out: 'Starting about 1960, the modern techniques of analytical chemistry, especially chromatography, provided the possibility to detect more and more dope agents or their metabolites in biological fluids, preferably in urine'.[22] A fundamental problem was that doping continued to be associated with professional sport. The IOC in particular was determined to maintain the amateur/professional distinction. It would take another highly public sporting death in 1967 before the IOC took any significant anti-doping action.

In 1967, British cyclist Tommy Simpson died during the Tour de France. Although initially attributed to heart failure from heat exhaustion, lack of oxygen and humidity, amphetamines, methylamphetamine and cognac were found in Simpson's body. In addition, traces of amphetamine were found in Simpson's jersey pockets and drugs were found in his luggage.[23] Simpson's death was not the only doping related death that year, with two cyclists, Belgian Roger de Wilde and Spaniard Valentin Uriona, both dying from amphetamine use. What was significant about Simpson's death was that it was the first *televised* doping death.

The television coverage of Simpson's death, as well as the impending 1968 Mexico Olympics, added a sense of urgency to the IOC's anti-doping efforts. Despite passing numerous resolutions condemning doping in the 1960s the IOC did not establish a formal Medical Commission until *after* Simpson's death.[24] At this time the IOC adopted new regulations requiring all Olympic athletes to pledge they would not use PESM, to submit to medical sex examinations,[25] and agreed to establish a medical centre at the 1968 Mexico Olympics to check 'for the use of dope and other stimulants'. At this time, the IOC defined doping as:

> The use of substances or techniques in any form or quantity alien or unnatural to the body with the exclusive aim of obtaining an artificial or unfair increase of performance in competition.[26]

The IOC also developed a list of prohibited substances and adopted a Medical Code.[27] Nevertheless, doping continued and athletes 'talked freely not about the morality of taking drugs, or the danger of being caught, but of practicality: which drugs were most effective'.[28]

In 1968, the first IOC drug tests found nothing more than alcohol use. Heavier testing at the 1972 Munich Games caught seven athletes using banned drugs including ephedrine and amphetamines. Consequently, many SGBs felt that routine, random testing had brought doping under control. However, these results demonstrated that one of the effects of anti-doping regulations was that athletes would look to a wider range of drugs to avoid detection. The emergence of anabolic steroids showed that athletes simply used drugs which were either absent from the banned list or as yet detectable (see the section on 'The history of drug testing in sport' for more on this important point).

In 1968, the list of banned substances did not include steroids and tests looked only for non-steroidal drugs. This was despite increasing steroid use during the 1950s and 1960s. For example, in 1956, more than 10 years before the IOC introduced testing in 1968 and long before testing for steroids commenced, Olympian Olga Fikotova Connally said: 'There is no way in the world a woman nowadays in the throwing events, at least the shot put and the discus, can break the record unless she is on steroids. These awful drugs have changed the complexion of track and field'.[29] In the late 1950s, United States physician Dr John Ziegler gave Dianabol to three weightlifters and within a short period of time steroids spread from sport to sport. It was clear that both Soviet and American athletes were using either male hormones or steroids to increase power and strength.[30] However, steroids were not added to the IOC banned list until detection technology became available in 1973.

Demonstrating again that detection and testing spurred the discovery of new ways to dope, athletes replaced steroids with testosterone. At the time, it was virtually impossible for the testing procedures to distinguish between naturally occurring testosterone and artificial or exogenous testosterone.[31] According to Houlihan, as 'many as two thirds of all random urine samples contained abnormal levels of testosterone' at the 1980 Moscow Olympics.[32]

Complicating anti-doping efforts in the 1970s and 1980s was the political climate of the Cold War. In this context, sporting performances were essential to national prestige and ideological supremacy. This situation has been described as a 'performance arms race' between the United States and the Soviet Union.[33] The reaction of SGBs to PESM during the period of the Cold War took different forms. In the socialist nations, such as Eastern bloc European countries, steroid use was institutionalized by governments and sports federations. For example, according to a 1973 *Le Monde* article:

> The East German doctors are said to have developed undetectable drugs. These are widely used for scientific purposes... Treatment with anabolic steroids has been generalised, together with the introduction of male hormones for girls, even for the very young.[34]

While SGBs in western nations, such as the United States, took a public anti-drug stance, they have also been accused of blocking effecting drug testing programmes or covering up positive tests results.

While the Cold War had drawn to a close by the end of the 1980s, it would be inaccurate to say that East German doping technology disappeared as the communist state dissolved. Rather, as Hoberman points out, 'it has been migrating to hospital research and sports programs around the world'.[35] Furthermore, the perception that doping was confined to specific sports, countries or events was an obstacle to anti-doping efforts. For example, high levels of steroid use were reported in weightlifting, powerlifting, body building, professional football and the throwing events in track and field.[36] As Houlihan notes: 'The popular perception within sport was that doping was, at worst, a manageable irritation, and certainly not a central responsibility of the International Federations or their domestic affiliates'.[37]

As we have seen, there are many historical precedents which illustrate that doping in sport is not a new phenomenon. Throughout the early twentieth century, the question of whether or not PESM *could* be used in sport was answered affirmatively. However, from the 1960s, the health risks associated with PESM use raised the issue of whether these substances *should* be used. Increasing numbers of sporting deaths, and in particular those which attracted significant media and public attention, acted as a catalyst for the development of anti-doping policies and procedures.

We should not – The push towards anti-doping in the 1990s

The philosophical underpinning of contemporary anti-doping policies is that PESM threaten athletes' health.[38] This is augmented by the claim that PESM use is unfair as it allows doped athletes to 'cheat' by surpassing 'natural' performance levels.[39] According to the Fédération Internationale de Football Association (FIFA), to be effective anti-doping must 'protect our players from harm and ensure that they can compete on equal grounds'.[40] The preamble to the IOC Olympic Charter against Doping in Sport states:

> That the use of a doping agent is both unhealthy and contrary to the ethics of sport, and that it is necessary to protect the physical and spiritual health of athletes, the values of fair play and competition, the integrity and unity of sport, and the rights of those who participate in it at whatever level.[41]

Combined with concern for athletes' health and equality of competition, athletes who use PESM are also argued to be bad role models for young people.[42] Consequently, SGBs at the local, national and international levels implemented anti-doping policies in their code of practice.[43]

However, athletes continue to use a range of PESM. These include steroids, human growth hormone (hGH), erythropoietin (EPO), insulin, ephedrine and amphetamines, as well as a number of other substances.[44] In addition, the risks associated with PESM continue to be highlighted. For example, the deaths of 18 cyclists between 1987 and 1990 are believed to be linked to EPO use.[45]

As doping continues despite the introduction of anti-doping policies, the legitimacy of SGBs has come under attack. MacAloon and Hoberman[46] argue that a significant factor contributing to the current doping problem is that the IOC no longer enjoys 'legitimacy'. The efforts of SGBs to address doping have also been criticized. For example, UK Athletics was accused of undermining anti-doping following the appointment of Linford Christie[47] as a mentor to Britain's sprinters.[48] Similarly, the world swimming organization, Fédération Internationale De Natation (FINA), was criticized for its 'failure to make even the most tentative gesture to keep drugs from our sport'.[49] However, a significant doping scandal in 1998 prompted SGBs and the IOC as well as governments to take action.

Just as highly public deaths in the 1960s drove anti-doping efforts, a highly public incident in the 1998 Tour de France provided impetus for anti-doping work. The scandal unfolded as a *soigneur* (a massage therapist and general assistant to cyclists) with the Festina cycling team was caught by customs officers with large amounts of EPO and hGH.[50] The significance of these events was pointed out by Hoberman, who stated that: 'The 1998 Tour de France doping scandal transformed the politics of doping by revealing that an entire athletic community – athletes trainers, physicians, and officials – had been practicing and concealing comprehensive doping as a way of life'.[51] In the wake of continuing doping scandals, drug testing has become central to the legitimacy of sport. For this strategy to be effective requires internationally uniform rules, policies, enforcement and sanctions.[52] However, when the 1998 Tour de France scandal hit, this uniformity was lacking.

WADA: twenty-first century anti-doping

Accordingly, and in response to the Tour de France doping scandal, the IOC convened the 1999 World Conference on Doping in Sport.[53] In turn, this conference led to the creation of the World Anti-Doping Agency (WADA) representing a partnership between the IOC, the sports movement and governments. One of the most significant tasks facing WADA is the harmonization of sports doping policies.[54] The enormity of this task cannot be overstated.

While the IOC is the Olympic governing body, SGBs establish and maintain the rules of their individual sports. As a result, there are more than 50 sets of rules governing the use of drugs in sports as well as differences between national and international competitions.[55] The situation is further complicated by some SGBs being reluctant to pass authority to other organizations. For example, FIFA argues that neither the IOC nor WADA has the right to dictate the terms of disciplinary action or doping sanctions.[56]

Nevertheless, WADA is committed to furthering the anti-doping ideology. In 2004 WADA introduced the World Anti-Doping Code (WADC) to ensure uniformity of rules and regulations, irrespective of the sporting context.[57] According to Richard Pound, WADA Chairman, the organization is determined to:

> Do all that we can to level the playing field and protect the spirit of sport. Our commitment to the fight against doping in sport has never been stronger, and we are dedicated to advancing research, monitoring and ensuring worldwide compliance with the Code, continuing the development of anti-doping programs, and facilitating the distribution of information and education for athletes and their entourage.[58]

To facilitate government support for WADA, the International Intergovernmental Consultative Group on Anti-Doping in Sport (IICGADS) was established in 1999 to coordinate and harmonize governmental action.[59] The significance of IICGADS was the creation, for the first time, of a global forum for governments to exchange views on doping and to coordinate governments' contribution to WADA.[60]

WADA called upon governments to begin the process of harmonizing their domestic policies with the WADC. The initial step in this process was the signing of the Copenhagen Declaration – the political document indicating government's commitment to the WADC and which now has 183 signatories.[61] This was followed by the drafting of an International Convention under the umbrella of the United Nations Education, Science and Cultural Organisation (UNESCO), providing governments with the practical means of harmonizing domestic policies with the WADC. The International Convention against Doping in Sport was unanimously adopted in October 2005 by the 191 countries participating in the UNESCO General Conference in Paris and came into force on 1 February 2007.[62]

WADA continues to expand its role and is intensifying efforts to target not only PESM-using athletes, but also those who facilitate and encourage doping. To accomplish this task, WADA coordinates investigatory work with SGBs as well as multiple government agencies such as customs, drug and law enforcement agencies.[63] According to WADA Director General David Howman:

> We want to get to a position where an investigatory body, operating under its national laws, can work alongside and cooperate with sports authorities so that sports can proceed with the sports sanctions in a timely manner while government authorities enforce laws relating to the supply and manufacture of doping substances.[64]

Some thoughts on the history of drugs in sport

When he revived the Olympic Games in 1896, Baron Pierre de Coubertin called on the unwritten rules of 'fair play' and emphasized participation with the motto that: 'The most important thing in the Olympic Games is not winning but taking part. The essential thing in life is not conquering, but fighting well'.[65] At the same time, however, the Olympic motto '*Citius, Altius, Fortius*' (faster, higher, stronger) places increasing pressure on the individual athlete to succeed. Athletes increasingly face pressure from both the media and the public to maintain performance levels. For example, even after securing a bronze medal at the 1960 Rome Olympics, American high jumper John Thomas stated:

> They only like winners. They don't give credit to a man for trying. I was called a quitter, a man with no heart. American spectators are frustrated athletes. In the champion, they see what they would like to be. In the loser, they see what they actually are, and they treat him with scorn.[66]

When doping controls were first implemented in the 1960s it was assumed that comprehensive drug testing and strict sanctions would eliminate doping. The strong motivation of athletes to reach the top of their profession demonstrates this is a poor assumption.[67] Despite the efforts of governments,

SGBs, the IOC and WADA, doping continues to be an issue in sport. For example, despite nearly 40 years of various anti-doping efforts, 2006 seemed to witness a new high profile doping scandal every month, including Tour de France cyclist Floyd Landis and Olympic sprint champion Justin Gatlin testing positive for abnormal ratios of testosterone to epitestosterone.[68]

Elite athletes are constantly evaluated based on their results and in an environment in which victories and records are linked to financial and social rewards, the temptation to use PESM can be difficult to resist.[69] For example, Jacobs and Samuels report Goldman's 1984 survey, which asked 198 athletes whether they would take a drug that would guarantee them a gold medal, knowing they would die in five years – 52% said yes.[70] If this is the state of affairs at the elite level, it is somewhat frightening to speculate what might be happening at the semi-professional or recreational levels.[71] In such a context, neither fierce crackdowns nor legalisation are likely to solve the historically deep problems of doping in sport. As Carstairs argues, it is questionable whether anti-doping strategies will achieve anything without accompanying social changes to the emphasis attached to success and winning.[72]

The history of drugs in sport: a working knowledge

At this point readers have a sound working knowledge about the background to drugs in sport, without being too in-depth. Importantly, the historical evolution explains a lot about why drugs in sport have gone in certain directions. A key idea is that drugs have been a part of enhancing human performance for a long time. More importantly, the reason for the change in the tolerance for drugs in sport seems largely confined to the second half of the twentieth century.[73] It would appear that the largely biochemical question of whether drugs *could* be refined and manufactured for the purpose of performance enhancement has been answered with a resounding 'yes'. On the other hand, there is still some question about whether those drugs *should* be used for performance enhancement, especially in the context of sport. Detailed commentary is deferred as this question is explored throughout the book.

As argued strongly above, one of the factors that influences the '*should*' is whether athletes can be caught. It is one thing to have an anti-doping policy and ban a substance, and another for that policy to be implemented for athletes who violate the policy. This makes it important to know about what happened to the implementation of anti-doping policies through the science behind detecting PESM use.

A brief history of drug testing in sport

The purpose of this section is to introduce the reader to the history of some of the PESM used by athletes in terms of the development of tests to detect their use. This is well short of a lesson about the complex chemistry underlying the drugs used in sport and their detection.[74]

The responsibility for developing tests capable of detecting prohibited PESM rests with WADA accredited laboratories. This reactive approach allows athletes a window of opportunity to use a drug without fear of being caught; the prospect of 'gene doping' means this window may be permanently open (see below). The main thrust of the argument behind this brief history of drug testing is based on the idea that drug testing laboratories are generally required to play catch-up, behind the scientists who create, and the athletes who use, performance enhancers.

Stimulants

The stimulants that athletes use typically fall into the broad categories of substances that include caffeine (methyl xanthines), adrenalin/ephedrine, amphetamines and cocaine.[75] The reason athletes take stimulants is because they 'increase the rate, and hence the work capacity, of the heart, central nervous system, and respiratory system'.[76] Athletes consuming stimulants increase their risk of injury, heat-stroke, psychosis or cardiac arrest.[77] While stimulants do have an effect on performance, the gains variably depend on the type of sport, especially in relation to caffeine.[78]

The use of stimulants in sport has been acknowledged with evidence that the use of 'pep pills' by soccer (football) teams in the UK was commonplace in the 1920s.[79] Through the Second World War, soldiers were given amphetamine-like substances to enhance mental awareness and offset fatigue.[80] As noted in the section, Brief history of drugs in sport, concerns about the use of stimulants in sport heightened with the death of Olympic cyclist Knud Jensen in 1960, and were reinforced by the televised death of Tour de France cyclist Tommy Simpson in 1967. These as well as other doping events led to the introduction of testing for stimulants at the 1968 Mexico summer and Grenoble winter Olympic games, even though it was known that athletes were using steroids.[81] This was an important milestone for drug testing in sport and represented the first active step in detecting drug use by athletes across the spectrum of nations and sports.[82] The testing for stimulants to the exclusion of other substances (steroids) continued at the 1972 Munich summer and Sapporo winter games.[83] Thus, it took about eight years to develop a test once it became apparent stimulants were having a negative impact on sport.

Anabolic-androgenic agents

The early 1950s saw a more potent drug family, anabolic-androgenic agents, being used for performance enhancement by athletes.[84] Anabolic-androgenic agents are synthetic derivatives of the hormone testosterone.[85] This synthetic testosterone is used for its anabolic (aids in metabolizing protein and muscle building) and androgenic (the part of testosterone that makes males male) qualities, and is commonly referred to as 'anabolic steroids'.[86] George[87] reports mixed evidence of steroids improving athletic performance in terms of gaining muscle mass, aerobic performance or improved muscle repair. George also suggests the benefit may lie outside the building of muscle mass, and may lie instead with increased lean body mass for runners or increased aggressiveness for rugby, American football or ice hockey.

During the 1972 Munich games, track and field athlete Jay Sylvester unofficially polled all male track and field athletes and found that 68% reported using some form of anabolic steroid.[88] In 1973 British scientists reported the successful development of reliable tests for anabolic steroids using radioimmunoassay (RIA) and gas chromatography and mass spectrometry (GC-MS).[89] During the 1976 Montreal/Innsbruck Olympics, testing for anabolic steroids was introduced using RIA (first sample) and GC-MS for confirmation (using the second sample) of any positive result. At the 1980 Moscow Olympics the GC-MS screen was unofficially used to test testosterone use by athletes based on the ratio of testosterone to epitestosterone (the T/E ratio).[90] Epitestosterone is a naturally occurring hormone that is similar to testosterone except for the orientation of one atom.[91] Where the T/E ratio is normally 1:1, use of testosterone can increase this ratio with 6:1 being suspicious and 10:1 indicating plausible guilt.[92] This leads to epitestosterone being used as a masking agent for synthetic testosterone by keeping the ratio low. In 1983 the T/E ratio test was first officially used at the Pan American Games in Caracas with a number of athletes testing positive and speculation being raised about several others who had either performed well below standard or had withdrawn from competition.[93] It seems to have taken about 11 years to develop a reliable test for steroid use that had an impact on athletic participation and performance.

Erythropoietin[94]

Synthetic erythropoietin (EPO) was understood to be in use by athletes from around the mid-1980s. Natural EPO is a substance important to erythropoiesis (the production of red blood cells) and controls how much blood is made and when. Athletes can use synthetic EPO to boost the amount of red blood cells their body makes, which means their body has more oxygen available and therefore increased capacity to sustain aerobic activity.[95] This makes it attractive to sports that require more than about one minute of sustained effort, and is particularly appealing to athletes in road cycling or long distance swimming. The main risk associated with EPO is elevated blood pressure when engaging in aerobic activity[96] and higher than normal blood viscosity (how thick the blood is), both of which increase the risk of heart failure.

Over the years a number of deaths have been directly attributed in cycling to the use of EPO and speculation exists that many more deaths could be attributed if autopsies had been performed. The Sydney Olympics in 2000 saw the first official test available for screening for EPO use, although this test has come under scrutiny in relation to its reliability. Despite this, WADA has decreed that a positive urine test for EPO is acceptable evidence of abuse.[97]

Human growth hormone

Human growth hormone (hGH) has been known to be used by bodybuilders since the early 1980s, and was also reported that athletes in the 1984 Los Angeles Olympics were using GH.[98] The use of hGH allegedly became so commonplace at the 1996 Atlanta Olympics that they were referred to as the 'Growth Hormone Games'.[99] The science behind how hGH works is rather complex as it interacts with a range of other hormones to produce different effects.[100] At its basic level, hGH promotes protein accretion (conversion of proteins to build muscle), muscle fibre hypertrophy (existing muscles get bigger) and improves muscle performance.[101] George[102] notes that abuse of hGH can lead to diabetic symptoms, elephant dermis (where the skin is too thick for standard gauge syringe needles), skeletal changes (e.g. enlarged fingers and toes) or enlargement of the heart (cardiomegaly; which can kill hGH abusers). George goes on to report that children may abuse, or be abused with, hGH to achieve the height or weight requirements of some sports (such as wrestling, volleyball or basketball). The consequences of an adolescent abusing hGH for simplistic or short term goals could be psychologically and psychiatrically catastrophic in the longer term, especially if the adolescent fails to achieve in the desired sport.

To the date of writing there is no reliable test to determine if an athlete is abusing hGH.[103] The problem for detection-based deterrence is a combination of ignorance about what is considered a normal level (such as the T/E ratio) and what would constitute a level that results in an unfair performance advantage.[104]

Gene doping[105]

Gene doping is the popular expression for using the science of genetics to influence the perform ance of athletes. According to Munthe there are four main ways genetics can influence athletes:

1. Fine tuning drugs to athletes on the basis of genetic profiling (genomics);
2. Changing, for example, blood cells to improve endurance (somatic cell modification);
3. Changing the genetic structure of embryos (germ line modification);
4. Choosing athletes on the basis of their genetic profile (genetic selection).

Having said this, gene doping is a different class of problem for a discussion on drugs in sport because the technology to use genetics in these ways is yet to be developed to a point it would have any practical effect.[106] Unlike other performance-enhancing drugs, Miah suggests there is an opportunity to develop policy and tests in parallel with the development of 'gene doping'; meaning there would be no gap between the two. That is, unlike other forms of doping, gene doping may be fully regulated before it becomes an issue. Of course the issue is rather more complicated philosophically and scientifically than has been presented here.

The window of opportunity

Technology and science has greatly improved athlete performance both legally (training, nutrition and biomechanics), and illegally (banned PESM). Technological advances have also meant that the scientists tasked with detecting these substances and methods are better equipped to do so. It is clear from the preceding discussion of even a few select substances that there is a window of opportunity for performance-enhancing substances or methods to be used by athletes between development or use and the capacity for detection. It is encouraging for the implementation of anti-doping policies that the window between drug use and drug detection has, with some exceptions, reduced over the years, possibly as a result of the increased focus placed on the drugs in sport issue by governments and SGBs. The significant consequence for scientists tasked with detection research is that they are reactive rather than proactive. Development of a test is usually a consequence of a new drug identified as performance enhancing and used by athletes to gain an 'unfair' competitive advantage (at least in Baron de Coubertin's sense). Of course, identifying which substances or methods athletes are using can be difficult as they are unlikely to advertise that they have been provided with a new drug.

This leads to a vexing question as to whether the National Anti-Doping Organisation (NADO) should be concerned that tests are unavailable for drugs that have been placed on the banned list. This issue is by no means a new one, as an American weightlifter pointed out in 1969, 'They couldn't pick it up in the test they were using. When they get a test for that one, we'll find something else. It's like cops and robbers'.[107] This highlights that the dilemmas faced by NADOs and drug testing laboratories have changed little over the history of drug testing in sport. It seems that banning a substance before a test is available may do nothing more than undermine the credibility of the system and make anti-doping policies the proverbial toothless tiger.[108]

The history of drug testing in sport: a working knowledge

Where the history of drugs in sport led from the question of 'could' to 'should', the history of drug testing in sport takes the implementation of anti-doping policy from 'should' to 'could'. That is, writing anti-doping policies is only one aspect of the complexity associated with drugs in sport; implementing those policies through testing is another layer of complexity that may never be resolved.[109] Of course, WADA and NADOs are just as aware of the potential failure to implement anti-doping policies through drug testing (e.g. GH or gene doping). This awareness has seen an evolution in anti-doping that creates a solid basis to argue the case for social science and drugs in sport: the transition from detection- to prevention-based deterrence.

The case for social science

As has been argued in the histories, the method of choice to achieve doping-free sport has largely been based on weeding out athletes who sought some kind of unfair advantage from using performance enhancing substances or methods. This means finding out if an athlete is using a prohibited substance or method based on some kind of medical test. In more technical language, the dominant strategy that characterized anti-doping during the twentieth and early twenty-first centuries was to reduce demand for PESM through detection-based deterrence.[110] Let us look more closely at what is meant by deterrence and detection in this context.

Deterrence in this context seeks to achieve some ideology in relation to sport by 'deterring' certain kinds of behaviours. An example of the ideology of sport can be seen in the WADC 'Spirit of Sport' statement,[111] which identifies what a range of experts say participation in sport is supposed to be about. The statement provides some insight into the behaviours desirable and hence promoted in sport (e.g. fair play and fun) and which behaviours are undesirable and need to be deterred.

The method of detection to achieve deterrence of at least drug behaviours follows the logic behind the medical model of dealing with illness. In its simplistic short form, the medical model seeks to determine which symptoms can be traced back to a pathogen which then indicates the type of treatment required. For example, a runny nose and a cough might be the symptoms of a cold. The cold is caused by some pathogen. The treatment for this pathogen is perhaps some pharmaceutically advised cold remedy, a nice chicken soup and some rest.

When deterrence and detection are conjoined, the model that results can be readily applied to the sporting context. In this case diagnosing the symptoms that lead to performance, or how well the athlete has been doing. Anti-doping is interested in whether the pathogen (or cause) of performance comes from natural talent and hard work, or some kind of prohibited enhancement. Detection then means identifying those who 'dope' and excluding them from competition for a violation of the governing set of rules to which participants must subscribe.[112] The theoretical effectiveness of this model follows the logic that an increased probability of detection and sanction leads to decreased use.[113]

The approach taken to anti-doping is more complicated than has been represented here; but the basic logic remains. Catch the athletes who cheat, make an example of them and everyone else will see sense and stop using. This logic relies on the assumptions that the tests reliably catch athletes and that testing actually deters athletes.

As noted in the history of drug testing, there has been a historical time lag between the development of new detection methods and new drugs that avoid detection, creating something of an arms race of drugs in sport.[114] The time lag between the invention of new drugs or methods and the ability to detect them is decreasing, which means identifying more users. Unfortunately, there are some substances that defied detection for years (e.g. steroids); moreover, detection-based deterrence could be facing an impasse with the rise of gene doping for which there may never be a reliable test. This means that the anti-doping ideology is faced with the significant problem of being unable to diagnose the pathogen of performance as natural or something added to the genetic structure at some point after conception.[115] So the first assumption of detection indicates that while it is possible to reliably identify some users, the chances of detecting all users is less than perfect and has the potential to decline rapidly.

The second assumption points to detection actually deterring athletes from using. It only takes a short glance at sports media to determine the deterrence value of detection. As noted earlier, despite 40 years of detection-based anti-doping effort, 2006 saw a number of elite professional athletes test positive for prohibited substances, including cycling (Landis), athletics (Gatlin), rugby union (Sailor) and cricket (Akhtar). Based on this, it might be fair to say that the chance of getting caught (detection) *versus* the effect of performance enhancement seems to be a risk that athletes are willing to take. In other words, while detection may deter some athletes it equally fails to deter others.

So it seems that detection-based deterrence may have reached its limit, and may start waning as a good way of dealing with drugs in sport.[116] If detection-based deterrence has indeed reached its limit as a deterrent for drug use by athletes, it is time to consider alternative deterrent strategies.[117]

Prevention-based deterrence

When confronted with a new problem like this, the philosophy of science suggests going back to first principles to reconstruct the ideas using a different approach. The first principle of relevance is that of deterrence discussed above. The second question is establishing why there is a concern about drugs in sport at all. This question has been answered, in part, by the history of drugs in sport, in the sense that people started dying from using performance-enhancing drugs. At the start of the twenty-first century, drugs in sport were specifically identified as contrary to what sport is supposed to be about (the WADC 'Spirit of Sport' statement) and therefore something to be deterred. This is formalized by the anti-doping stance advocated by the IOC and implemented by WADA and NADOs. Right or wrong, the anti-doping stance was the dominant ideology driving drugs in sport research at the time of writing. The ideology says, therefore, that the goal is to achieve drug-free sport.

The medical model, as it has been used thus far, refers to deterring athletes from using prohibited substances or methods through detection. Another way of describing detection-based deterrence using the language of the medical model is that it is a form of 'secondary prevention'. Secondary prevention refers to the idea of treating or curing some one after they have fallen sick. That is, preventing a pathogen from making people even more gravely ill with treatment. In this case, the pathogen is drugs in sport and it is treated by excluding athletes who have used in an effort to protect the rest of sport, the same way a surgeon might cut away cancerous growths from one part of the body to stop cancer from spreading. The concern here is treating the pathogen that exists without necessarily being concerned with the reasons the pathogen turned up in the first place. That is, the aim of secondary prevention is to treat and hopefully cure the existing ailment. So detection-based deterrence might be seen as a way of curing drugs in sport.

The medical model recognizes that treatment is only half of the story. Once the person has been treated and cured of their ailment, it is better for them to avoid getting that illness again. This follows the idea of 'it hurts when I do this; well stop doing that!' It is also useful for other people to know that 'it hurts when I do this, so you probably want to avoid it too'. That is, stopping the pathogen before it starts. This implies a different kind of prevention called primary prevention. The main concern here is identifying how to prevent the need for treatment in the first place or to instil the idea that prevention is better than cure. Applying the idea of primary prevention to sport means achieving drug-free sport by stopping athletes from taking drugs in the first place, or deterring drug use by stopping it before it starts. Translating from the medical model, this could be called prevention-based deterrence.

Working towards effective prevention-based deterrence means looking into the world of the athlete to work out what influences drug use in sport. Pausing to consider what might influence drugs in sport provokes a number of questions about how the personality of an athlete might make them more likely to use prohibited enhancers, or how the big money associated with sport might promote drug use in sport. Such questions have the character of issues social science attempts to answer.

Does social science have anything to offer?

The framework that guided deeper consideration of whether social science has anything to offer prevention-based deterrence was based around how the individual, the group and the organization/institution might influence drugs in sport.

The individual

A striking question at this level of consideration is why an athlete might use a performance enhancing substance or method. The most obvious answer to this question is 'to win', but this might be an oversimplification of the issue. For example, an athlete might take a prohibited substance on the orders of their coach, to ensure they get a bonus for the number of matches they play each year, appearance fees, or just to remain competitive against a younger crop of players.[118] This suggests that the reasons for taking prohibited enhancers might be more sophisticated than 'to win'.[119] Changing direction, it might be equally worthwhile to find out just how much work prevention-based deterrence has to do by establishing how many athletes are influenced by detection-based deterrence. Answering these questions seems germane to psychology or economics.

The group

Taking one step back from the athlete, it is readily apparent that athlete drug use may be influenced by those around them; which suggests questions on the social network of the athlete.[120] The first element of the social network that may be worth asking about is the support staff, the team that prepares the athlete for competition such as their coach, sports physician, nutritionist or physiotherapist. While support staff may be influential for the elite level athlete, family or friends might be more influential for the aspiring or non-elite athlete. This all suggests that it might be important to know how support staff, friends or family are themselves influenced in relation to the use of performance-enhancing substances or methods. For example, ambitious parents might be easily persuaded by a well-meaning coach and introduce a contaminated supplement into the diet of a young athlete. Looking at this level suggests understanding drug use by athletes may be the result of combined efforts by people other than just the athlete. Prevention-based deterrence therefore requires some insight into how the people around the athlete might influence drug use. Again, there is a set of questions that could be answered using methods from the social sciences, especially sociology.

The institution

Taking another step further back from the athlete is how institutions influence drug use. Institutions can be the club athletes play for, the organizations that run the competition, the media or betting agencies, the medal aspirations of a nation, or which sport attracts the most spectators. Prevention at this level means understanding what incentives exist for institutions to make sure their sports are drug free. The IOC does this by excluding cities whose countries fail to sign on to the WADC (explicitly included in both the Questionnaire for Applicant and Candidate Cities). One consequence of this might mean the sport or country in question misses out on the chance to take part in the Olympics. An important question is working out what makes an institution choose one way or the other. This set of ideas places us firmly in the realm of social science, as they specifically address how social organizations interact to produce changes in human behaviour.

At an even more abstract level, the evidence we collect in relation to answering such questions may take us one step back from the anti-doping stance. In the anti-doping context, prevention-based deterrence means getting athletes to abstain from using prohibited substances or methods for their entire sporting careers. The evidence collected from researching prevention-based deterrence may inform whether the anti-doping stance is a good one to take. For example, the deterrence issue could disappear if the rules change and drugs in sport are permitted. Even if this does happen, the prevention-based deterrence research effort will inform how athletes think about performance and competition, and also performance enhancement as part of the human condition in relation to non-sport activities (e.g. cosmetic surgery or Viagra).

Returning to the question at hand: *does social science have anything to offer prevention-based deterrence?* The above makes a case that social science has a lot to offer. Unfortunately, there is no steady or coordinated stream of social science research into drugs in sport. This journal aims to help address this by pointing out areas in need of attention by social science. The areas needing attention are systematically analysed and reported to define an agenda to guide research by social scientists (or anyone else for that matter) into this field of inquiry.

Notes

1 This observation, made by Bøje, is reported in Hoberman, *Mortal Engines.*

2 For example, the British Medical Association advocates for more social science based research in BMA, *Drugs in Sport.*

3 This history of drugs in sport draw on several key references, including Donohoe and Johnson, *Foul Play*; Hoberman, *Mortal Engines* and 'Sports Physicians and the Doping Crisis in Elite Sport'; Ordway, 'Drugs in Sport'; Stokvis, 'Moral Entrepreneurship and Doping Cultures in Sport'; Todd and Todd, 'Significant Events in the History of Drug Testing and the Olympic Movement: 1960–1999'; and, Verroken, 'Drug Use and Abuse in Sport'. In the interests of endnote brevity, unless otherwise stated, assertions of historical fact or interpretation can be ascribed to one of these sources.

4 McArdle, '"Say it Ain't So, Mo"', and Miah, 'From Anti-doping to a "Performance Policy" Sport Technology, being Human, and doing Ethics'.

5 International Olympic Committee, *Olympic Movement Anti-Doping Code*, 6.

6 Birchard, 'Past, Present, and Future of Drug Abuse at the Olympics'.

7 Ibid., 1008; and Crowther, 'The Salt Lake City Scandals and the Ancient Olympic Games'.

8 Crowther, 'The Salt Lake City Scandals', 170.

9 Kennedy, 'Newer Drugs Used to Enhance Sporting Performance'; Ordway, 'Drugs in Sport'.

10 Cashmore, *Making Sense of Sports*; Yesalis, Kopstein and Bahrke, 'Difficulties in Estimating the Prevalence of Drug Use among Athletes'; Kennedy, 'Newer Drugs Used to Enhance Sporting Performance'; Ordway, 'Drugs in Sport'.

11 Donohoe and Johnson, *Foul Play*, 4. Linton was reported to have died in 1886, during the Bordeaux to Paris race, after having apparently been given an overdose by his trainer. However, Linton won the Bordeaux to Paris race and, according to *The Cycling World Illustrated*, died in July 1896 of what was diagnosed as typhoid fever. The British Cycling Federation notes that Linton was one of several riders trained by a particular coach and that a number of these riders were given strychnine during competition. While the cause of Linton's death was apparently typhoid fever, it is likely that he was doped and that, in the long-term, this may have contributed to his ill-health and subsequent death.

12 Drug Think, 'The Doping Scandal: A Question for Sport'.

13 See Hoberman, *Mortal Engines*, 6.

14 See Hoberman, '*Sports Physicians*', 204.

15 Cited in Yesalis, Kopstein and Bahrke, 'Difficulties in Estimating the Prevalence of Drug Use among Athletes', 44.

16 Jacobs and Samuels, 'The Drug Testing Project in International Sports', 562; Ordway, 'Drugs in Sport', 17.

17 See Donohoe and Johnson, *Foul Play*; and Ordway, 'Drugs in Sport'.

18 Houlihan, 'The World Anti-Doping Agency: Prospects for Success', and Stokvis, 'Moral Entrepreneurship and Doping Cultures in Sport'.

19 Dyreson, *Making the American Team*, 39.

20 Since renamed the International Association of Athletic Federations.

21 Bowers, 'Abuse of Performance-enhancing Drugs in Sport'.

22 Cited in McArdle, '"Say it Ain't So, Mo"', 92.

23 See Cashmore, *Making Sense of Sports*; and Giulianotti, *Sport: A Critical Sociology.*

24 Derived from ASADA's, 'History of Drugs in Sport', http://www.asada.org.au/antidoping/history.htm; and McArdle, '"Say it Ain't So, Mo"', 92–3.

25 It was widely believed at the time that the practice of men pretending to be women to compete in women's events was prevalent. According to McArdle, '"Say it Ain't So, Mo"', in approximately 30 years of sex testing at athletic events no case was ever documented. Interestingly, it was only after her death in 1980, that Stella Walsh – winner of 41 AAU titles and two Olympic medals – was found to be a man (Donohoe and Johnson, *Foul Play*).

26 Cited in Todd and Todd, 'Significant Events in the History of Drug Testing and the Olympic Movement: 1960–1999', 68.

27 See Bowers, 'Abuse of Performance-enhancing Drugs in Sport', and Giulianotti, *Sport: A Critical Sociology*.
28 See Cashmore, *Making Sense of Sports*, 110.
29 Cited in Wright and Cowart, *Anabolic Steroids: Altered states*, 3.
30 See ASADA, 'History of Drugs in Sport'.
31 See McArdle, '"Say it Ain't So, Mo"', 94.
32 Houlihan, *Dying to Win*, 71.
33 Bahrke and Yesalis, 'The Future of Performance-enhancing Substances in Sport'; Drug Think, 'The Doping Scandal'; and Jacobs and Samuels, 'The Drug Testing Project in International Sports', 559.
34 Cited in Brohm, *Sport: A Prison of Measured Time*, 20.
35 See Hoberman, *Mortal Engines*, 226 and 228.
36 See Yesalis, Kopstein and Bahrke, 'Difficulties in Estimating the Prevalence of Drug Use among Athletes'.
37 Houlihan, 'The World Anti-Doping Agency: Prospects for Success', 125.
38 WADA, *World Anti-Doping Code.*
39 See Jacobs and Samuels, 'The Drug Testing Project in International Sports', 558–9.
40 Blatter, 'FIFA's Commitment to Doping-free Football', i1.
41 See Drug Think, 'The Doping Scandal'.
42 Carstairs, 'The Wide World of Doping: Drug Scandals, Natural Bodies, and the Business of Sports Entertainment'; Ordway, 'Drugs in Sport'; and, Yesalis, Kopstein and Bahrke, 'Difficulties in Estimating the Prevalence of Drug Use among Athletes'.
43 See Bowers, 'Abuse of Performance-enhancing Drugs in Sport', and McArdle, '"Say it Ain't So, Mo"'.
44 See Yesalis, Kopstein and Bahrke, 'Difficulties in Estimating the Prevalence of Drug Use among Athletes'.
45 Hoberman, *Mortal Engines*, 2–3; and Parisotto, *Blood Sports*, 36.
46 MacAloon, 'Doping and Moral Authority: Sport Organisations Today', and Hoberman, 'How Drug Testing Fails: The Politics of Doping Control'.
47 Christie, who won the Olympic 100 meters gold medal at the 1992 Barcelona Olympics, tested positive for nandrolone in 1999 and was banned for two years.
48 Agencies report at http://www.theage.com.au/news/sport/gold-medal-tainted-by-drugs/2006/08/07/1154802822652.html.
49 Leonard, 'Doping in Elite Swimming: A Case Study of the Modern Era from 1970 Onward', 229.
50 See MacAloon, 'Doping and Moral Authority: Sport Organisations Today'; Voet, *Breaking the Chain*, xi; and, Waddington, *Sport, Health and Drugs*, 155–9.
51 See Hoberman, 'How Drug Testing Fails: The Politics of Doping Control', 264.
52 See Jacobs and Samuels, 'The Drug Testing Project in International Sports', 580 and 588.
53 See MacAloon, 'Doping and Moral Authority: Sport Organisations Today', 205–6.
54 Mendoza, 'The War on Drugs in Sport: A Perspective from the Front-line'; Miah, 'From Anti-doping to a "Performance Policy" Sport Technology, being Human, and doing Ethics'.
55 See Bowers, 'Abuse of Performance-enhancing Drugs in Sport'; and Ordway, 'Drugs in Sport'.
56 Dvorak *et al.*, 'FIFA's Approach to Doping in Football'.
57 Gilberg, Breivik and Loland, 'Anti-doping in Sport: The Norwegian Perspective'.
58 WADA, 'Chairman's Message'.
59 See Houlihan, *Dying to Win*, 173.
60 Ibid.
61 See WADA, 'Chairman's Message'.
62 Ibid., and International Sports Movement, 'World Anti-Doping Agency WADA Executive Committee and Foundation Board Advance Closer to Final Revision of the World Anti-Doping Code'.
63 See International Sports Movement, 'World Anti-Doping Agency WADA Executive Committee and Foundation Board'.
64 See http://www.wada-ama.org/en/newsarticle.ch2?articleID=3115421.
65 Cited in Donohoe and Johnson, *Foul Play*, 128.
66 Ibid., 129.
67 See Houlihan, *Dying to Win.*
68 Commentary of Landis's drug test positive at the 2006 Tour de France from http://www.iht.com/articles/2006/07/27/sports/bike.php and http://www.telegraph.co.uk/sport/main.jhtml?view = DETAILS&grid = &xml = /sport/2006/09/13/socycl13.xml; and Gatlin's sanction from athletics at http://www.smh.

com.au/news/sport/gatlin-accepts-eight-year-ban/2006/08/23/1156012575477.html and http://sport.guardian.co.uk/athletics/story/0,1833820,00.html.

69 See Gilberg, Breivik and Loland, 'Anti-doping in Sport: The Norwegian Perspective'.

70 See Jacobs and Samuels, 'The Drug Testing Project in International Sports', 586–7.

71 A key issue facing the management of drugs in sport and the anti-doping policy is that no one really knows what the prevalence rates are at any level of sport.

72 See Carstairs, 'The Wide World of Doping'.

73 See Waddington, *Sport, Health and Drugs.*

74 Both Mottram, *Drugs in Sport*, and Bahrke and Yesalis, *Performance Enhancing Substances in Sport and Exercise*, are excellent sources of technical accounts on the chemistry and pharmacology of performance-enhancing drugs.

75 Kammerer, 'Drug Testing and Anabolic Steroids'.

76 Anshel, 'Drug Abuse in Sport: Causes and Cures', 418.

77 See Chapters 21–24 in Bahrke and Yesalis, *Performance Enhancing Substances in Sport and Exercise.*

78 George, 'Central Nervous System Stimulants'.

79 See Waddington *et al.*, 'Drug Use in English Professional Football'.

80 See Houlihan, *Dying to Win*; and Verroken, 'Drug Use and Abuse in Sport', 30.

81 The testing at the 1968 games was used to evaluate the efficacy of the tests and the testing procedure. Formal tests were introduced for the 1972 games (from Kammerer, 'Drug Testing and Anabolic Steroids'). See also Todd and Todd, 'Significant Events in the History of Drug Testing and the Olympic Movement: 1960–1999', for an account of when advances in drug testing influenced the development of anti-doping policy.

82 Beckett, Tucker and Moffat, 'Routine Detection and Identification in Urine of Stimulants and other Drugs'.

83 According to Ferstle, 'Evolution and Politics of Drug Testing', there was some limited testing by the Italian cycling and soccer federations in the 1950s and other sporting organizations in the early 1960s, although none matched the scale of that associated with the Olympic effort (see Todd and Todd, 'Significant Events in the History of Drug Testing and the Olympic Movement: 1960–1999').

84 George, 'Androgenic Anabolic Steroids'.

85 Yesalis, *Anabolic Steroids in Sport and Exercise.*

86 Bahrke and Yesalis, 'Anabolic-androgenic Steroids'.

87 George, 'Androgenic Anabolic Steroids'.

88 See Todd and Todd, 'Significant Events in the History of Drug Testing and the Olympic Movement: 1960–1999'.

89 Brooks, Firth and Sumner, 'Detection of Anabolic Steroids by Radioimmunoassay'.

90 See Kammerer, 'Drug Testing and Anabolic Steroids'.

91 See George, 'Androgenic Anabolic Steroids'.

92 Kammerer, 'Human Chorionic Gonadotropin'.

93 Todd and Todd, 'Significant Events in the History of Drug Testing and the Olympic Movement: 1960–1999', report that by failing to place in the event they were not required to provide a urine sample.

94 This section relies heavily upon the work of Parisotto, *Blood Sports*, and Armstrong and Reilly, 'Blood Boosting and Sport'. As in previous sections, a citation is noted only where sources other than these two are relied upon to support assertions about the nature of reality.

95 Yesalis *et al.*, 'Incidence of Anabolic Steroid Use: A Discussion of Methodological Issues'.

96 Ekblom, 'Erythropoietin'.

97 Verroken and Mottram, 'Doping Control in Sport'.

98 Yesalis and Bahrke, 'History of Doping in Sport'.

99 From Yesalis, Kopstein and Bahrke, 'Difficulties in Estimating the Prevalence of Drug Use among Athletes'.

100 See George, 'Peptide and Glycoprotein Hormones and Sport', or Kraemar, Nindl and Rubin 'Growth Hormone: Physiological Effects of Exogenous Administration', for sound technical accounts of hGH.

101 From Kraemar, Nindl and Rubin 'Growth Hormone: Physiological Effects of Exogenous Administration'.

102 See George, 'Peptide and Glycoprotein Hormones and Sport'.

103 See Verroken and Mottram, 'Doping Control in Sport'.

104 See Kammerer, 'Human Chorionic Gonadotropin'.

105 This section relies upon Munthe, 'Selected Champions: Making Winners in an Age of Genetic Technology', and Miah, *Genetically Modified Athletes*. The latter is a comprehensive examination of the issues surrounding gene doping.

106 Although Durmanov, 'Discussion on the Present Challenges and Issues for the Fight against Doping and where Scientific Knowledge would Help', argues otherwise.

107 Gilbert, 'Drugs in Sport: Problems in a Turned On World', 66.

108 See Ferstle, 'Evolution and Politics of Drug Testing', 369–70.

109 See Houlihan, 'The World Anti-Doping Agency: Prospects for Success'.

110 Ibid.

111 WADA, *World Anti-Doping Code*.

112 Ibid.

113 See Anshel, 'Drug Abuse in Sport: Causes and Cures'.

114 See Bahrke and Yesalis, 'The Future of Performance-enhancing Substances in Sport'.

115 Winning an arbitrary contest of human mind, body and/or spirit is so important to some they might consider genetically modifying humans to achieve sporting success. This has been the mainstay of horse racing through selective breeding. As an extension of the selective horse breeding idea, Miah, *Genetically Modified Athletes*, raises the unsettling question of what to do with the children of genetically modified athletes.

116 Houlihan, 'Anti-doping Policy in Sport: The Politics of International Policy Co-ordination'; and, Laure *et al.*, 'Drugs, Recreational Drug Use and Attitudes towards Doping of High School Athletes'.

117 See BMA, *Drugs in Sport*; and Houlihan, *Dying to Win*.

118 See Waddington, *Sport, Health and Drugs*.

119 See Houlihan, *Dying to Win*.

120 See BMA, *Drugs in Sport*.

References

Anshel, M.H. 'Drug Abuse in Sport: Causes and Cures'. In *Applied Sport Psychology: Personal Growth to Peak Performance*, 4th ed., edited by J.M. William, 416–44. Mountain View, CA: Mayfield Publishing Company, 2001.

Armstrong, D.J., and T. Reilly. 'Blood Boosting and Sport'. In *Drugs in Sport*, 4th ed., edited by D.R. Mottram, 207–27. USA: Routledge, 2005.

Bahrke, M.S., and C.E. Yesalis. 'The Future of Performance-enhancing Substances in Sport'. *The Physician and Sports Medicine* 30, no. 11 (2002): 51–3.

Bahrke, M.S., and C.E. Yesalis. *Performance Enhancing Substances in Sport and Exercise*. Champaign, IL: Human Kinetics, 2002.

Bahrke, M.S., and C.E. Yesalis. 'Anabolic-androgenic Steroids'. In *Performance Enhancing Substances in Sport and Exercise*, edited by M.S. Bahrke and C.E. Yesalis, 33–46. Champaign, IL: Human Kinetics, 2002.

Beckett, A.H., G.T. Tucker, and A.C. Moffat. 'Routine Detection and Identification in Urine of Stimulants and Other Drugs, Some of which may be Used to Modify Performance in Sport'. *Journal of Pharmacy and Pharmacology* 19 (1967): 273–94.

Birchard, K. 'Past, Present, and Future of Drug Abuse at the Olympics'. *The Lancet* 356 (2000): 1008.

Blatter, J.S. 'FIFA's Commitment to Doping-free Football'. *British Journal of Sports Medicine* 40, Suppl. 1 (2006): 1.

BMA. *Drugs in Sport: The Pressure to Perform*. London: BMJ Publishing Group, 2002.

Bowers, L.D. 'Abuse of Performance-enhancing Drugs in Sport'. *Therapeutic Drug Monitoring* 24 (2002): 178–81.

Brohm, J.-M. *Sport: A Prison of Measured Time*. London: Ink Links, 1978.

Brooks, R.V., R.G. Firth, and N.A. Sumner. 'Detection of Anabolic Steroids by Radioimmunoassay'. *British Journal of Sports Medicine* 9 (1975): 89–92.

Carstairs, C. 'The Wide World of Doping: Drug Scandals, Natural Bodies, and the Business of Sports Entertainment'. *Addiction Research and Theory* 11, no. 4 (2003): 263–81.

Cashmore, E. *Making Sense of Sports*, 4th ed. Abingdon: Routledge, 2005.

Crowther, N. 'The Salt Lake City Scandals and the Ancient Olympic Games'. *International Journal of the History of Sport* 19, no. 4 (2002): 169–78.

Donohoe, T., and N. Johnson. *Foul Play: Drug Abuse in Sports*. Oxford: Blackwell, 1986.

Drug Think. 'The Doping Scandal: A Question for Sport'. DrugScope, 2004. http://www.drugscope.org.uk/about/project_hometemplate.asp?id=55.

Durmanov, N. 'Discussion on the Present Challenges and Issues for the Fight Against Doping and where Scientific Knowledge would Help'. Paper presented at the Conference on Ethics and Social Science Research in AntiDoping, Larnaca, Cyprus April 2006.

Dvorak, J., T. Graf-Baumann, M. D'Hooghe, D. Kirkendall, H. Taennler, and M. Saugy. 'FIFA's Approach to Doping in Football'. *British Journal of Sports Medicine* 40, Suppl. 1 (2006): 3–12.

Dyreson, M. *Making the American Team: Sport, Culture, and the Olympic Experience*. Urbana, IL: University of Illinois Press, 1998.

Ekblom, B.T. 'Erythropoietin'. In *Performance Enhancing Substances in Sport and Exercise*, edited by M.S. Bahrke and C.E. Yesalis, 101–8. Champaign, IL: Human Kinetics, 2002.

Ferstle, J. 'Evolution and Politics of Drug Testing'. In *Doping in Elite Sport: The Politics of Drugs in the Olympic Movement*, edited by W. Wilson and E. Derse, 363–413. Champaign, IL: Human Kinetics, 2001.

George, A.J. 'Central Nervous System Stimulants'. In *Drugs in Sport*, 4th ed., edited by D.R. Mottram, 64–102. New York: Routledge, 2005.

George, A.J. 'Androgenic Anabolic Steroids'. In *Drugs in Sport*, 4th ed., edited by D.R. Mottram, 140–90. New York: Routledge, 2005.

George, A.J. 'Peptide and Glycoprotein Hormones and Sport'. In *Drugs in Sport*, 4th ed., edited by D.R. Mottram, 191–206. New York: Routledge, 2005.

Gilberg, R., G. Breivik, and S. Loland. 'Anti-doping in Sport: The Norwegian Perspective'. *Sport in Society* 9, no. 2 (2006): 334–53.

Gilbert, B. 'Drugs in Sport: Problems in a Turned On World'. *Sports Illustrated* June 23 (1969): 66.

Giulianotti, R. *Sport: A Critical Sociology*. Cambridge: Polity Press, 2005.

Hoberman, J. *Mortal Engines: The Science of Performance and the Dehumanisation of Sport*. USA: The Blackburn Press, 1992.

Hoberman, J. 'How Drug Testing Fails: The Politics of Doping Control'. In *Doping in Elite Sport the Politics of Drugs in the Olympic Movement*, edited by W. Wilson and E. Derse, 241–74. Champaign, IL: Human Kinetics, 2001.

Hoberman, J. 'Sports Physicians and the Doping Crisis in Elite Sport'. *Clinical Journal of Sport Medicine* 12 (2002): 203–8.

Houlihan, B. 'Anti-doping Policy in Sport: The Politics of International Policy Co-ordination'. *Public Administration* 77 (1999): 311–34.

Houlihan, B. *Dying to Win*, 2nd ed. Strasbourg: Council of Europe Publishing, 2002.

International Olympic Committee. *Olympic Movement Anti-Doping Code*. Lausanne: International Olympic Committee, 2000.

Houlihan, B. 'The World Anti-Doping Agency: Prospects for Success'. In *Drugs and Doping in Sport Socio-legal Perspectives*, edited by J. O'Leary, 125–45. London: Cavendish Publishing Limited, 2001.

International Sports Movement. 'World Anti-Doping Agency WADA Executive Committee and Foundation Board Advance Closer to Final Revision of the World Anti-Doping Code'. *Sports Features Communications*, 14 May 2007. http://www.sportsfeatures.com/index.php?section=pp&action=show &id=39088

Jacobs, J.B., and B. Samuels. 'The Drug Testing Project in International Sports: Dilemmas in an Expanding Regulatory Regime'. *Hastings International and Comparative Law Review* 18, no. 3 (1995): 557–89.

Kammerer, R.C. 'Drug Testing and Anabolic Steroids'. In *Anabolic Steroids in Sport and Exercise*, 2nd ed., edited by C.E. Yesalis, 415–59. Champaign, IL: Human Kinetics, 2000.

Kammerer, R.C. 'Human Chorionic Gonadotropin'. In *Performance Enhancing Substances in Sport and Exercise*, edited by M.S. Bahrke and C.E. Yesalis, 323–39. Champaign, IL: Human Kinetics, 2002.

Kennedy, M.C. 'Newer Drugs Used to Enhance Sporting Performance'. *Medical Journal of Australia* 173, Special Olympic issue (2000): 314–7.

Kraemar, W.J., B.C. Nindl, and M.R. Rubin. 'Growth Hormone: Physiological Effects of Exogenous Administration'. In *Performance Enhancing Substances in Sport and Exercise*, edited by M.S. Bahrke and C.E. Yesalis, 65–78. Champaign, IL: Human Kinetics, 2002.

Laure, P., T. Lecerf, A. Friser, and C. Binsinger. 'Drugs, Recreational Drug Use and Attitudes Towards Doping of High School Athletes'. *International Journal of Sports Medicine* 25 (2004): 133–8.

Leonard, J. 'Doping in Elite Swimming: A Case Study of the Modern Era from 1970 Onward'. In *Doping in Elite Sport: The Politics of Drugs in the Olympic Movement*, edited by J. Wilson and E. Derse, 225–39. Champaign, IL: Human Kinetics, 2001.

MacAloon, J.J. 'Doping and Moral Authority: Sport Organisations Today'. In *Doping in Elite Sport: The Politics of Drugs in the Olympic Movement*, edited by J. Wilson and E. Derse, 205–24. Champaign, IL: Human Kinetics, 2001.

McArdle, D. '"Say it Ain't So, Mo". International Performers' Perceptions of Drug Use and the Diane Modahl Affair'. In *Drugs and Doping in Sport Socio-Legal Perspectives*, edited by J. O'Leary, 91–108. London: Cavendish Publishing, 2001.

Mendoza, J. 'The War on Drugs in Sport: A Perspective from the Front-line'. *Clinical Journal of Sport Medicine* 12 (2002): 254–8.

Miah, A. 'From Anti-doping to a "Performance Policy" Sport Technology, Being Human, and Doing Ethics'. *European Journal of Sport Science* 5, no. 1 (2005): 51–7.

Miah, A. *Genetically Modified Athletes: Biomedical Ethics, Gene Doping and Sport*. UK: Routledge, 2004.

Mottram, D.R. *Drugs in Sport*, 4th ed. New York: Routledge, 2005.

Munthe, C. 'Selected Champions: Making Winners in an Age of Genetic Technology'. In *Values in Sport: Elitism, Nationalism, Gender Equality, and the Scientific Manufacture of Winners*, edited by T. Tannsjo and C.M. Tamburrini, 217–31. London: E & FN Spon, 2000.

Ordway, C. 'Drugs in Sport'. *The Law Society of South Australia Bulletin*, November 1998.

Parisotto, R. *Blood Sports: The Inside Dope on Drugs in Sport*. Prahran, VIC: Hardie Grant Books, 2006.

Stokvis, R. 'Moral Entrepreneurship and Doping Cultures in Sport'. *ASSR Working Paper Series 03/04*, November 2003.

Todd, J., and T. Todd. 'Significant Events in the History of Drug Testing and the Olympic Movement: 1960–1999'. In *Doping in Elite Sport: The Politics of Drugs in the Olympic Movement*, edited by W. Wilson and E. Derse, 65–128. Champaign, IL: Human Kinetics, 2001.

Verroken, M. 'Drug Use and Abuse in Sport'. In *Drugs in Sport*, 4th ed., edited by D.R. Mottram, 29–63. New York: Routledge, 2005.

Verroken, M., and D.R. Mottram. 'Doping Control in Sport'. In *Drugs in Sport*, 4th ed., edited by D.R. Mottram, 309–56. New York: Routledge, 2005.

Voet, W. *Breaking the Chain. Drugs and Cycling: the True Story*. London: Yellow Jersey Press, 2001.

WADA. *World Anti-Doping Code*. Montreal: World Anti-Doping Agency, 2003.

WADA. 'Chairman's Message'. WADA. http://www.wada-ama.org/en/dynamic.ch2?pageCategory.id=254.

Waddington, I. *Sport, Health and Drugs: A Critical Sociological Perspective*. London: E & FN Spon, 2000.

Waddington, I., D. Malcolm, M. Roderick, and R. Naik. 'Drug Use in English Professional Football'. *British Journal of Sports Medicine* 39, no. 18 (2005).

Wright, J.E., and V.S. Cowart. *Anabolic Steroids: Altered States*. Carmel, IN: Cooper Publishing Group, 1990.

Yesalis, C.E. *Anabolic Steroids in Sport and Exercise*, 2nd ed. Champaign, IL: Human Kinetics, 2000.

Yesalis, C.E., and M.S. Bahrke. 'History of Doping in Sport'. In *Performance Enhancing Substances in Sport and Exercise*, edited by M.S. Bahrke and C.E. Yesalis, 1–20. Champaign, IL: Human Kinetics, 2002.

Yesalis, C.E., A.N. Kopstein, and M.S. Bahrke. 'Difficulties in Estimating the Prevalence of Drug Use among Athletes'. In *Doping in Elite Sport: The Politics of Drugs in the Olympic Movement*, edited by W. Wilson and E. Derse, 43–62. Champaign, IL: Human Kinetics, 2001.

Yesalis, C.E., M.S. Bahrke, A.N. Kopstein, and C.K. Barsukiewicz. 'Incidence of Anabolic Steroid Use: A Discussion of Methodological Issues'. In *Anabolic Steroids in Sport and Exercise*, 2nd ed., edited by C.E. Yesalis, 73–115. Champaign, IL: Human Kinetics, 2000.

Debating the role of drugs in sport: a reader

Jason Mazanov

School of Business, UNSW@ADFA, Canberra, Australia

The development of the agenda to guide social science research into drugs in sport was driven by two workshops. The first workshop examined basic drugs in sport issues, and attempted to put a common lexicon or discourse to frame and explore different ways of thinking about the issues. Development of this framework saw a first principles approach built from the purpose of social science towards the questions that proved starting points to understanding the issues at hand. The second workshop challenged the academic approach to drugs in sport with a hypothetical scenario discussed by people involved in the sports industry, including athletes, policy makers and parents of athletes. The results of these workshops form an insight into one attempt of a multi-disciplinary group to come to grips with how social science can contribute to relevant social issues such as understanding the role of drugs in sport.

The little research into drugs in sport using social science methods that does exist is both sporadic and isolated.[1] One way of resolving the sporadic and isolated nature of this research towards steady and coordinated social science research is to develop a reference point from which social science can explore drugs in sport phenomena. In this sense, the development of the agenda serves the purpose of planting a flag so that social science can get some indication of where it has been and where it can go.

The team that worked on the agenda came from across the social sciences spectrum, including economics, educational psychology, health psychology, law, sociology and sport philosophy. This dynamic mix of disciplines enabled the team to achieve the cosmopolitan research agenda reported later in this collection. Another important characteristic of the team was the combination of established researchers in the field of drugs in sport with social scientists for whom the topic was novel. In this sense the team had a mix of those published in the field and others coming to the topic 'fresh'.

The work which eventually led to the agenda was developed over the course of two workshop meetings and almost 12 months of continuous research effort. The first workshop, held in February 2006, aimed to provide a common body of knowledge for the team, such that those for whom drugs in sport was a novel topic could get 'up to speed' relatively quickly. The second workshop, held in July 2006, looked to develop an integrated and collaborative approach to social science research of drugs in sport phenomena.

A note

The current essay looks at some of the issues arising from the workshops as context for the other parts of the collection. Reporting on the creative output of so many people who spend their lives looking for new ways of seeing the world was daunting for the author, with so many ideas deserving of a line of research in their own right. Since this essay effectively reports several long and in-depth conversations, readers are encouraged to reflect on how they would have approached the same issues. The aim here is for readers to agree or disagree with what the team came up with. If readers agree or disagree there is scope to do research by continuing the conversations from these workshops in the broader discussion of drugs in sport.

The first workshop

In the first workshop the team identified two sets of questions that helped scope what 'drugs in sport' means. The first set of questions arose out of the team's general discussion of drugs in sport using the philosophical framework presented by Dr Dennis Hemphill. The second set of questions (derived from the first) was our initial discussion (led by Professor Stephen Mugford) on what social science could do to inform the drugs in sport debate. Both sets were seen as sound basic questions to ask in trying to work out how social science can engage with drugs in sport phenomena. The team felt that these questions represented a good place to start for anyone looking to develop their understanding of drugs in sport issues, especially those concerning social science.

The first set of questions

When a science is confronted with an issue that has received little consideration, the appropriate starting point is to ask basic questions, such as definition. The team looked to answer the question about what social science needs to research to better understand drugs in sport using three guiding ideas. The *first idea* was defining the social contexts relevant to drugs in sport phenomena. The *second idea* represented the observational component of the scientific method. The model proposed to guide observation at this early stage of research into drugs in sport using social science methods was 5W analysis, or 'who, what, when, where and why' (proposed by Dr Keiran Sharpe). Such observations are meaningless without transforming the data into information through evaluation. This led to the *third idea* where observations are analysed to determine whether there are any themes or stories that might become the basis for theory. That is, developing theory from the ground up by looking at the way things work (deductive) instead of trying to predict them using logic (inductive).

Social context

The discussions commenced with a clarification of the analytic framework of social science by defining what was meant by social. This discussion established that the social context had to be limited to 'sport', making the definition of sport crucial. There are already many contrasting views about what characterizes sport,[2] and it is well outside the scope of this essay to discuss what sport means in detail. Some common elements that seem to emerge across these definitions suggest that, at a general level at least, sport involves some set of *skilled activity* that is organized into a *structured competition*. Of course, these two ideas mean just about any organized test of skill can be defined as sport. To get a better sense of what a sport is, the general understanding of sport follows those recognized by the International Olympic Committee (IOC). This leads to some vexing questions, such as the status of chess as a sport, but sufficed for the broad ranging discussion pursued in the workshops.

Identifying the social contexts within sport that may influence the use of performance enhancing substances and methods (PESM) becomes a very important part of the definitional process. Social science arguably uses three basic units of analysis for social phenomena: the individual, the group and the institution or organization. Each of these units is analysed by variation within (intra) and between (inter).

The individual level of analysis concentrates on what drives an individual to do something (variation within the individual or 'intra-individual'), or the behaviour of one individual relative to another (variation between individuals or 'inter-individual'). An example of this is a sport psychiatrist helping a triathlete overcome depression. The group level of analysis looks at what happens when enough individuals come together towards some level of cooperative activity. This includes how individuals behave within the group context (intra-group behaviour) as well as how they behave relative to another group (inter-group behaviour). This might be characterized by a sport psychologist helping a water polo team sort out their differences to believe they can compete equally with other teams. The institutional or organizational context relates to the collection of groups with a common purpose. For example, the Fédération Internationale de Natation (FINA) organizes and administers all the different swimming federations across the world for international competition.[3] The intra-institutional activity might be looking at how they set up rules for 'clean' competition, and inter-institutional activity might be how they interact with the government hosting an international swimming championship.

As the team discussed these social contexts, one issue that appeared to constrain our thinking was the assumption that any conversation on drugs in sport referred only to elite or professional athletes. While the elite or professional level is where the issue of drugs in sport is most prominent (e.g. media sensation) and has the greatest consequence (e.g. stripping of medals, suspensions or bans), 'non-elite' athletes are just as important to a social science of drugs in sport. For example, adolescent males seem to be particularly vulnerable to using protein supplements, some in their efforts to become elite athletes.[4] Another example is the social hockey player who uses creatine to gain an edge over other social players.[5] The use of drugs at any level of sport (junior, senior, social, amateur, elite or professional) is of central interest to social scientists. If any notion from this collection shapes the future of drugs in sport research using social science methods, it must be that research into drugs in sport is never confined to the study of elite or professional level athletes.[6]

5W analysis

As a caveat to the following discussion, the examples given under the discussion of 5W analysis are by no means the only ones, nor are the interpretations of the 5Ws the best way of thinking about them. Examining these questions is designed to be a starting point for discussing drugs in sport issues using social science methods with an intention to be illustrative rather than authoritative. Readers are encouraged to discover better ways of thinking about the 5Ws than the interpretations offered here.

Who

The issue of 'who' seems to be one that is easily answered – the athletes, irrespective of their elite or non-elite status. This is a reasonable place to start before considering who else influences athlete's decision to use PESM.[7] That is, looking at who in the social network of athletes might be involved. The social network, or 'sportsnet' of the athlete is rather extensive, including coaches, trainers, physiotherapists, sports physicians, massage therapists, administrators, managers, other athletes, friends outside athletics, parents and even fans.[8] This list varies significantly depending on their level of competition (e.g. a junior social player is unlikely to have much contact with fans). This becomes even more complex when each of these groups is extrapolated beyond the individual to the group (e.g. the team) or the institutional level (e.g. national sporting organizations, sponsors, pharmaceutical companies, gambling organizations or the media).

At the institutional level, it is possible to start asking questions about who is interested in the prevention and the promotion of drugs in sport. This question led the team to suggest research that 'follows the money' for drugs in sport. Sport in the twenty-first century is an entertainment commodity that commands large amounts of money and resources.[9] Asking 'who makes money out of drugs in sport?' may be an important question for social science to address in examining drugs in sport phenomena.

An example of the complexity of the question 'who' is obvious in the medical ethics literature, alive with debate over the role of the sports physician and the general practitioner in PESM use by athletes. Some argue steroid use under the supervision of a qualified medical practitioner is a safer way of using such substances than independent use by the unqualified with substances of questionable quality. The same sort of debate is needed in relation to coaches or other support staff – do coaches and support staff need specialist training in the handling of substances like steroids to minimize the harm they may do? The problem here is that there is very little systematic research on what coaches or the support staffers actually do in relation to such supervision.

What

Looking at what athletes are using (in the case of substances) or doing (in the case of the methods) could give some insight into the drugs in sport issue. Studying the patterns of who uses what could become very important. Social science has already uncovered meaningful differences between the users of different kinds of drugs.[10] There is no reason to expect that drugs in sport would work any differently. For example, beta-blockers decrease the heart rate and lower anxiety,[11] which is great for sports like shooting but probably result in a performance decrement in basketball. Another example of this is the systematic use of 'social' (e.g. alcohol) or illicit drugs (e.g. ecstasy; 3-4 methylenedioxymethamphetamine) to help an athlete recover from the psychological rigours of competition more rapidly than other athletes. It is possible to argue that an artificially improved recovery may lead to subsequent performance that could be attributed to drugs rather than natural talent. This would be entirely impractical to administer and enforce, but does represent an interesting question for ethicists and policy writers to consider.

What a drug is used for could vary on whether it is about improving performance (better than natural) or overcoming a performance decrement (allowing an athlete to reach their natural potential). For example, an athlete may suffer abnormal anxiety during competition to the point they have an anxiety disorder. To be put on an equal playing field with other athletes who have no anxiety disorder the athlete is prescribed a drug that brings their anxiety back to a 'normal' level for competition. That is, they are overcoming a performance decrement such that their natural talent can be expressed in competition. So using a social drug is clearly unnecessary for overcoming the potential decrement of psychological distress, the issue is a bit more difficult when psychological or psychiatric disorders are considered.

Knowing 'what' could also give some insight into the pressures (e.g. the need for strength) and vulnerabilities (e.g. feelings of inadequacy) that face athletes. An extension of the 'what' question for athletes is what sorts of drugs coaches feel are important to the success of their athletes. Developing a profile of coaches' list of drugs in sport preferences could be just as important as developing the profiles for athletes.[12] If this process is reiterated across people within a sport, it may be possible to develop a profile that informs an assessment of the performance-enhancing drug or substance use culture within that sport.

When

The question of 'when' can be asked in two ways. The first looks at when athletes use various drugs, usually dictated by the pharmaceutical properties and effects of PESM. For example, in altitude training, use of erythropoietin (EPO) or blood doping has to be timed to ensure it has the desired performance enhancing effect.[13] The second question of when asks when the risk of using banned substances or methods goes from unacceptable to acceptable. Individual analysis of athletes, parents or coaches could provide valuable insight into the turning point when natural talent is no longer enough, or sport goes from *ludic* (the notion of playing for the sake of play) to competition.[14] These questions can also be extrapolated to the group. For example, the team winning may become more important than playing or competing, or indeed the health and wellbeing of any individual team member.[15] The institutional level raises this to an even more concerning extreme. For example, when does the profit motive become more important than the long-term quality of life of the athlete?

Where

Looking at the issue of 'where' in terms of the three social contexts (individual, group and organizational) suggests social science research could start with where individuals purchase the substances or methods, where users hide behind the group, and identifying where substances are made (organizational/institutional). At the individual level, a person can purchase prohibited substances, whether the athlete, the coach, support staff or parents, over the Internet, which may provide different messages of legitimacy of PESM purchase to images of illegal substances being traded under a veil of secrecy. At the group level, 'where' prohibited substances are used could also influence implied legitimacy; injecting steroids or blood doping at a sporting academy is very different to injecting in a back alley. Use at a sports academy may give users a sense that the group (the coach, the support team or the academy) is somehow condoning the use. At the institutional level is the question of 'where' the drugs come from, another way of 'following the money'. This becomes extremely pertinent when considering where new masking agents or new 'undetectable' drugs are being developed and distributed.

Why

To a degree, this is the question of most interest to social science. The use of substances or methods implies some degree of decision-making by someone at some level. For the individual this is a question of why they are using. The simple answer is 'to win'. This obvious explanation has to contend with research into other drug behaviour that shows the motivation to use a substance is rarely caused by one thing. For example, suggesting teenagers start smoking because of 'peer pressure' ignores other important influences like parental smoking, stress or self-esteem.[16] Other factors that might influence the use of PESM might include performance anxiety, sustaining a career for as long as possible or image enhancement. At the group level, it becomes important to understand why a sport has a particular predisposition to drug use. For example, comparing cycling as the standout sport with a long history of drug use with other Olympic sports that have a less obvious relationship. If differences do exist, it might help work out how to make cycling more like a drug resistant sport (if such a sport exists).[17] At the organizational/institutional level, the why question immediately points to ideas of why drug use in sport is so abhorrent when it is condoned in so many other aspects of human society. Of all the questions in the 5W analysis why is probably the one that is most attractive, yet it can only be meaningfully approached with serious research answering the other four 'W's.

The use of drugs in human society is remarkably prevalent, especially in relation to improving performance in specific contexts. A classic example of this comes from caffeine consumption in the industrialized West. Caffeine is a known stimulant, commonly used to improve performance (increase alertness) or overcome a performance decrement (tiredness). Another commonly used social drug is alcohol, often used to enhance (lubricate) social situations. At another level, the use of beta-blockers by elite classical musicians to reduce anxiety and steady their hands extends beyond an isolated few.[18] Even these cursory examples suggest that drug based performance enhancement is very much a part of human existence, which leads to the question of why a special case is made for the socially created (artificial) context of sport?

A note on the 5Ws

As noted earlier, the interpretation of the 5Ws represents some ideas that are immediately apparent to just one person. In writing this section, a decision was made to keep things superficial rather than delving into intricacies. For example, asking 'when' an athlete goes from being a non-user to a user is a very different take to the rather more concrete interpretation of 'when' used above. This could be extended to ask 'what' changes athletes from non-user to user, as opposed to the prevalence approach discussed. Developing a research agenda is about asking questions and, more importantly, working out which are the right ones to ask. So, if the reader has used the 5W discussion or approach to come up with their own questions, this section has achieved its purpose.

Theory building from the ground up

Once social science has some answers about the various social contexts using the 5Ws, theory building can begin. Theory building is usually conducted top-down (a sequence of logical propositions or argument) or bottom-up (based on observations of reality and attempting to identify common patterns apparent in those observations). The approach taken by the team was to focus more on the bottom-up approach to develop theory grounded in the reality that has already been observed. The description of drugs in sport phenomena using the 5W approach would provide social scientists with a range of information needed to develop theory.

Importantly, there may be observations or evidence from similar phenomena that can be extrapolated to the drugs in sport *milieu*. For example, there has been a huge effort to understand substance use and abuse in terms of theory and results right across the social sciences. The important question is whether the theory and results developed on the rest of society applies in the specific social context of drugs in sport; for example, asking whether the processes that govern the uptake of heroin use can be applied to the uptake of steroid use. Further, there may be some question whether the system of laws designed to regulate the use of narcotics in society more broadly is applicable to the drugs in sport context. Some might argue either case represents completely different situations and others that they are similar to the point of being interchangeable. These are important enough issues that simple agreement or assumption is insufficient and compels the need for objective evidence to respond one way or the other.

The second set of questions

The second set of questions put to the team aimed to stimulate discussion and to discover possibilities. Three questions the team felt were central to developing our understanding of drugs in sport from a social science perspective were agreed upon and responded to using a hybrid of the 'World Café' approach under the guidance of Professor Stephen Mugford. After agreeing on the questions the team formed tables of four. One person 'hosted' the table. Their role was to start the conversation off (like a good host or hostess) and record what people said. After a period of time, everyone except the host changed tables to engage in a new conversation. The host (again being a good host or hostess) related where the conversation had arrived and how it arrived there to their new guests and then invited the conversation to continue. Stimulating discussion allowed the team to find out what they thought about drugs in sport issues and to explore how those thoughts differed from others. This was, in part, to give the team a sense of where disciplines converged and where they explored the same ideas from different perspectives. The discussion also allowed the team to discover what sorts of research projects might be possible to answer some fairly tough questions about drugs in sport.

In relating the questions and highlighting in part the direction of the conversations it is the team's hope that the reader is inspired to build on their efforts by continuing the conversations. The questions were:

1. If prohibition of drugs in sport is the answer, what is the question? (hosted by Trevor O'Donnell);
2. With respect to drug use, how different is sport? (hosted by Vanessa McDermott);
3. How do we best understand the why/when/who of PESM use? (hosted by James Connor).

As can be seen, the team were very interested in questions that represent the basis for any investigation of human behaviour by a social science.

If prohibition of drugs in sport is the answer, what is the question?

The aim of this question was to turn the issue on its head; society seems to have arrived at an answer – prohibition. The team explored the reasons that might lead to the prohibition. When the team cycled through the 'conversations', several themes emerged that began the process towards making sense of the answer of prohibition.

There was a general consensus that the answer of prohibition had to do with upholding a value or ideal. This could be related back to the 'Spirit of Sport' statement made in the WADC as to why people participate in sport. That is, sport is about health, enjoyment, bettering ones-self and so on. This view of sport might be a romanticized view of what a society feels sport 'should' be rather than what it is. That is, society likes their athletes to be the best of everything considered valuable, perhaps in physical, psychological and social ways. This makes the cause of prohibition one of upholding a set of values, an integral part of organized society.[19] However, the question of why sport should be considered sacred and held to a higher morality than other aspects of society dogged the discussion. It was eventually proposed that prohibition, to a certain extent, has to be accepted on faith as what a society wants for sports.

An extension that seeks to move beyond faith is the belief that sport is a remedy for a variety of social ills, such as delinquency among youth (by giving them focus and teaching discipline) or population level health, and that PESM somehow contaminates the curative power of sport. Waddington[20] argues that this is a fantasy created by questionable research that was politically popular for a period through the mid- to late-twentieth century. Waddington provides compelling evidence and argument that sport has no effect on delinquent behaviour, nor does it yield any health benefit (in fact, the evidence suggests sport is bad for one's health due to the injuries associated with participation). This suggests that the prohibition could be based on a misinformed assumption.

Another popular argument for prohibition is the notion of creating a level playing field. The team was particularly scathing of this notion given the rather pronounced effect economic inequalities have on sporting performance. Wealthy nations can afford to have their athletes do nothing but train, and train with quite a stunning array of support.[21] For example, to get an elite athlete into a Commonwealth, Olympic or Championship event might take a sportsnet that includes a coach, an assistant coach, a specialist in biomechanics, a nutritionist, a physiotherapist, a sports medical practitioner, a podiatrist, a sport psychologist and a remedial massage therapist. There is a cost to retaining these people even before the equipment is taken into account. This is in contrast with athletes who have to work full time and may be unable to even access training facilities.[22]

The discussions could find no defensible reason for banning PESM. The conversations were peppered with arguments negated by a lack of meaningful evidence, being based on misinformation, or being mitigated by a more convincing counter-argument. The only compelling argument was that of faith. This suggested that the prohibition was the result of sport administrations needing to be seen to be doing something in line with a prevailing belief, such as zero tolerance policies in relation to the use of other drugs (e.g. narcotics like heroin). This discussion is reflected by the broader literature (popular and scholarly) which regularly exposes flaws in the philosophical underpinnings of the ban on drugs in sport.[23]

This broader debate, to which this collection seeks to contribute, sees the community becoming more educated and opinions changing. If beliefs change this may lead to a question of how anti-doping efforts need to evolve to maintain social currency.[24] This provides an area rich for social science to explore changing opinions and their effect on drugs in sport activity at the individual, group and organizational levels.

With respect to drug use, how different is sport?

Drugs of various forms have been used to enhance human performance over the course of human history.[25] Historically, medicine has used drugs or substances to enhance the immune system to overcome illness or disease. This use is fundamental to survival. PESM are also used in less fundamental contexts. A simple example of this is the prevalence of caffeine use to help wake people up or keep them going later in the day. Another relates to substances claimed to improve memory, or cognition-enhancing drugs, popular among students.[26] A popular performance enhancing method is cosmetic surgery. For some reason, society permits its citizens to use these substances or methods to gain some advantage over others, either real or perceived. This returns to the question of why sport has been singled out for special treatment in the form of a system which polices the use of substances or methods widely available to the rest of society.

The attempt to answer this question led the conversation to consider what makes sport so special that it needs such tight social rules. The first idea was that sport represents some sort of 'leveller' that allows humans to play or compete with each other. This may have been rooted in the *ludic* notion of organized sport, or in commercialized sport as a desire to create exciting contests between equally skilled individuals or groups.[27] Another important idea was that because society permits athletes to have a higher physical standard, an athlete must also be held to a higher moral standard in their public and private lives. That is, society expects athletes to exchange their ability to be held to a lower moral standard for a privileged position in society (fitness, wealth and celebrity). While this describes only the absolute elite level of sport, media driven perceptions of sport based on this elite level may mean the higher standard is applied to sport at other (social and amateur) levels as well.

The issue of money came up in deliberations focusing on the commercialized nature of sport. There has been significant financial investment into sport from both the private (usually through advertising or media rights) and public sectors (tax breaks or direct government funding to support a sport). This may promote the perception that athletes have an obligation to the sport and the public to abide by certain rules, conditions and standards. Private interests would want to ensure their brand was associated with something positive (e.g. drug free sport) to promote those interests, or to ensure they continue to receive funding from public sources (e.g. government grants or spectator revenue). Public interests have to be held in line with international conventions (e.g. the WADC), policy stances on drugs (e.g. the 'War on Drugs' or zero tolerance policies) or governments making funding available on the basis that certain rules, conditions or standards are adhered to.[28]

Sport is an agreed set of rules or laws that establishes the nature of the competition, from sideline throw-ins, to the weight of a bat, to what a competitor needs to do to compete at certain events. A person, group or country must submit to these rules if they want to participate in sport either as a player or a spectator.[29] The rules are set and controlled by private interests (e.g. international sports federations or advertising), government interests (e.g. promoting a particular ideology) or the public (e.g. voting with their feet as to what they want to play or watch). Sport is special because it is a segment of society that can be controlled, and whose participants can be controlled because they voluntarily submit to a set of rules.

Discussion of the question of why sport is so special came to no firm conclusions. It seems hypocritical to allow everyone other than sportspeople to use PESM. Talking about the reasons for this hypocrisy led us to again consider the idea that sport needs to be held separately (but not in isolation) to the rest of a society, perhaps via the romantic ideal. The reason for this separation of sport was because athletes claimed a special status in terms of health, wealth or celebrity. The driver for this could be the result of intervention by private interest, government political ideologies or the public. One reason advanced for the interest in intervention was because sport represents a segment of society that can be controlled. While the ideas presented make for a good start, they are by no means an end to discussing this issue. Readers are encouraged to think of other reasons why sport is held to a different standard to the rest of society on drug-related issues.

How do we best understand the why/when/who of PESM use?

This particular discussion explored why sportspeople use PESM in the first place. Some time was spent diagnosing the reasons underlying drug use in the sporting context, eventually settling on three main reasons thought to be reflections of the sporting world: restoring the body after an injury, coping with being an athlete, and expanding or improving performance (to win). This demonstrated that 'to win' was too simplistic an explanation and proposed a range of other influences (such as self-esteem or institutional pressures). Note that while 'to win' is an important part of the drugs in sport research process, it must be acknowledged that there are also other reasons that need to be considered in a sound analysis of the reasons underpinning the use of PESM in sport.

The discussion turned to explanations for how competition works as a way of understanding why athletes use. The level playing field argument became a focus for scrutiny, with a slightly different focus. The premise that sporting outcomes rely on very slight variations came to fore. At the elite level the difference between first and last place can be almost too small to perceive. For example, the difference between first and second place in a swimming event could be measured in milliseconds, simply too quick for humans to discern a difference in performance. This tells us that any slight improvement could have a tremendous influence (e.g. improving a 10-second 100-metre sprinter by 3% results in a 9.7 second run). Operating at the fringe of human ability therefore means that very small changes in initial conditions can have a huge impact on outcome. Drugs therefore give athletes an opportunity to control more of the variation in outcome.

This simple argument is an important intellectual exercise towards understanding the processes which govern athlete PESM use. The outcome of competition can be reconceptualized as a mathematically chaotic (non-linear) process, where theoretically the flapping of a butterfly's wings in Brazil can change the outcome of a world championship event in Osaka, Japan.[30] It is this apparently (linearly) unpredictable nature of competition that is attractive. For athletes this unpredictable nature is perhaps less desirable, as they want to maximize their competitiveness by making things as predictable and controlled as they can. That is, drug use is a form of risk management.[31] This leads to the attractive question of risk management for whom and for what?

Taking a more pragmatic line, the discussion turned towards looking at why athletes change their behaviour. For example, there could be very different reasons underlying why an athlete starts using, why they keep using, or why they stop using. Asking these sorts of questions of athletes might give a good insight into the sorts of things that need to be done to promote primary prevention. A consequence of such thinking was speculation about how far back intervention needs to be placed. It is one thing to have a set of factors informing work towards prevention-based deterrence and another to work out when the best time is to do it. As talent identification can occur at a very early age, does this mean that the prevention-based deterrence interventions also need to begin at that very early age? The answers to these questions could then be used as the basis for intervention programmes focused on what provokes changes in behaviour rather than describing the differences between behaviours.

While significant time was spent contemplating the sporting context, the notion of performance enhancing use more broadly was brought up. One example that was brought up was whether the factors underlying amphetamine use in a long haul truck driver were the same as those driving steroid use in athletes. This brought us to the much bigger question of what makes humans use any kind of PESM in the first place. There was a consensus that this was an important issue for drugs in sport research, and drugs research more broadly.

This discussion was important as a vehicle to think about what sport is and why drugs play a part in it in the first place. Importantly, 'to win' become one of a set of reasons athletes might use PESM rather than the only reason. This Café delivered a set of loosely related ideas that might serve as a basis for other deliberations on drugs in sport.

Some comments on the first workshop

The team came away from the first workshop with a sense of how much work social science needs to do. The combination of an intriguing problem with so much scope to do so many things provided confidence that developing a social science of drugs in sport was crucial towards a better informed debate on the issue.

The second workshop

The second workshop saw the team reconvene to build on the first. A significant amount of time was spent re-examining the questions raised in the first workshop with an eye to applying them to specific disciplines. There was a second World Café in which the team worked towards developing collaborative and cosmopolitan research in reference to some key questions reported in a later essay in this collection. In terms of reporting the second workshop, this left only one very important component that was appropriate to report here; the 'hypothetical' discussion.

The hypothetical

One characteristic of the team was a breadth of experience in social science, and perhaps less experience in the contemporary sport industry. The aim of this session was to get a different perspective on drugs in sport from the people who experience it as part of their everyday live.

A range of guests were invited to share their experience and understanding of drugs in sport, including:

- the parent of an emerging elite athlete;
- current elite athletes;
- a sports manager;
- a representative from Australia's national anti-doping organization (NADO) the Australian Sports Anti-Doping Authority (ASADA); and,
- a representative from the Australian Sports Drug Testing Laboratory (ASDTL).

Importantly, their contribution gives an indication of the difference between what policy or research proposes and what actually happens. The aim here was for the team and for readers of this collection to be a little more aware of the potential gaps between rhetoric and reality. One important gap already identified is the focus on elite athletes. The 'hypothetical' discussion gave the team pause to think about the reality for the non-elite or aspiring athlete, and how the rhetoric might be translated into reality for these people.

The scenario

The team members and invited guests were given the hypothetical situation outlined below as a starting point for discussing the experience of drugs in sport. The group was introduced to the mythical Kim and Jim.

> *Kim, Jim and the caffeine question*
> Kim and Jim are 15-year-old twins who have demonstrated significant talent for the same individual Olympic event. They are on the brink of national selection and have been in preparation for the next Olympics. There are a few events coming up that would really help their selection chances with some good performances and getting a bit more experience.
>
> Kim and Jim have come to you for some advice. They have been told that their chances of selection would improve if they got some 'extra help' in the form of a caffeine supplement. After a little probing and questioning, you learn that the product that has been recommended has had the occasional problem of being contaminated with prohibited substances.
>
> What advice would you give Kim and Jim, and why?
>
> As we consider the advice, also reflect on what sorts of things you don't know that you would like to know in giving advice to Kim and Jim.

Some ideas from the discussion

There were four key outcomes from the hypothetical discussion. Firstly, there was some advice on how to improve future scenarios. Secondly, there was a significant positive for the hard work currently done on educating athletes about drugs in sport. Thirdly, the issue of individual responsibility emerged as a big factor in the thinking on drugs in sport. This proved to be pivotal in our thinking and led to the fourth key learning point, which was the amount of trust in others athletes have to give in order to compete.

Note that due to the geographical location of the workshop the results are necessarily reflective of the Australian experience. Some observations are constrained to the Australian context, and others could be generalized beyond the Australian context.

Some advice for future scenarios

The role of scenario-based learning is an extension of the research agenda put forward for educational psychology. Readers wishing to run similar exercises in the future,[32] whether as part of an educational campaign or a research effort, can improve the design of their scenarios offered here. As the discussion evolved, it appeared that two characteristics of the hypothetical situation could be improved upon. The first was the issue of age, with the group suggesting that perhaps a brother and sister with one under the age of legal adulthood and one above might work better. The second was a suggestion that perhaps a substance other than caffeine may have provoked a different response from the group.

Knowledge

The role of education in relation to drugs in sport emerged as a significant positive where rhetoric and reality matched more than they differed. The athletes felt that they were provided a significant amount of information on the rules and regulations associated with implementation of the WADC. A technical interpretation of this is that the strategic intent of the WADC was achieving at least some alignment at the implementation level. That is, the efforts of the World Anti-Doping Agency(WADA) appeared to be having the desired effects on the people actually participating in sport. The sports managers were also complimentary of the education effort associated with drugs in sport. While there was no data on the effect of drugs in sport education from the country of origin (Australia), the response from the Café was supported by work conducted by UK Sport[33] in relation to the level of knowledge about anti-doping policy and procedures among elite athletes. The next step in terms of research is to determine whether the strategic intent of the WADC is also having the same effect at the non-elite levels, which is the main thrust of the discussion paper released by the Victorian Government.[34]

No one said 'don't'

Significantly, no one suggested that Kim or Jim should avoid using PESM. The general feeling of the group appeared to be that Kim and Jim had to make an informed choice about their use of a potentially-contaminated-but-otherwise-legal supplement. When probed, it appeared to be permissible to use caffeine as a PESM because it was absent from the prohibited list (at least in 2006). The implication (or at least the author's potentially incorrect interpretation) was that it is okay to use legal PESM despite their use being explicitly contrary to the WADC 'Spirit of Sport'. This raised an important set of the questions for the implementation of the 'drug free sport' ideology advocated by WADA. That is, the sports industry may be receiving mixed messages about PESM being a part of sport but only when they are permitted.

Another issue arising of the 'informed choice' path taken by the group is the notion of strict liability. Strict liability is the idea that if an athlete is caught with a prohibited substance in their body, they put it in knowing it was against the rules and are therefore sanctioned. At this point, however, it seems that the idea of strict liability may be influencing the perception that the fault and sanction lie entirely with the athlete. The group were more concerned with giving Kim and Jim advice on how to make an informed decision (e.g. education, or talking with experts; see below) in relation to the risks of using (e.g. performance benefit versus consequences of getting caught) rather than whether using is a good idea. This is another significant effect of the individual focus of strict liability potentially overlooking the role of the group or organization in drugs in sport phenomena.

While 'no one said don't', there were voices encouraging Kim and Jim to explore alternatives that might give them the performance enhancement they were looking for. The sports managers were adamant that Kim and Jim should look to a change in training, sleep patterns or diet to achieve the desired outcomes before they even consider resorting to what might be termed 'artificial' enhancement. Of course, Kim and Jim's response may be that such changes require more effort than taking a potentially contaminated supplement. This leads to questions about how athletes make decisions in relation to how they seek to improve their sporting performance.

The initial position of 'no one said don't' led to at least three practical ideas and potential avenues for research that may be initially obscured. The first was that there may be a rhetoric-reality gap in terms of 'drug free sport' and the acceptance that drugs are a part of sport. The second was that strict liability may be placing too much emphasis on the role of the individual athlete relative to other actors such as groups or organizations. The third idea was more insight is needed into how athletes actually make decisions about the manner in which they seek to improve their performance.

Trust

One theme from the discussion was that athletes are pretty busy people. Athletes (at least elite, professional and semi-professional) have to know more and more about how to train, cope with competing, what to eat when, recognizing minor and major injuries, the rules of their sport, how their sport is administered, what drugs do and the rules about drugs. In technical language, an athlete has to have a working knowledge of sport science, sport psychology, nutrition, sport medicine and the law for their particular sport; and then they have to actually participate in their sport. So, for an athlete to make an informed decision about something like using a PESM, they either have to know a lot or talk to other people. At the elite level, the athlete is effectively putting their career in the hands of some one else. At the non-elite level, the athlete could well be putting their health or their income in the hands of some one else. For athletes in general it means trusting other people.

Trust is a particularly difficult issue that has occupied the thoughts of philosophers and social scientists for a long time. Discussion of the technical aspects of trust are omitted in favour of looking at how it emerged in relation to Kim and Jim. Broadly speaking, there were two groups that Kim and Jim would probably turn to at this time for advice; experts and non-experts.

Experts, loosely speaking, are the people designated as some one an athlete can trust to know something about specialist areas. This might be some one with lots of certificates on their wall (e.g. medical practitioner, nutritionist or psychologist) or some one put in a position because of their experience giving them a level of expertise (e.g. a coach or sports administrator). The biggest issue for the discussion was that some experts may be well intentioned but misguided. For example, a general practitioner may have no idea that the patient consulting them is an athlete and may prescribe something on the prohibited list. Expecting general practitioners to be up-to-date on the prohibited list adds another burden to a medical specialization that already has a significant amount to contend with.[35] This is an error a sports medicine specialist is unlikely to make, although accessing such a specialist for a bout of influenza may be difficult and/or expensive. Similarly, a coach may be well intentioned in terms of wanting their protégé to succeed, but simply lack the specialist knowledge for drugs in sport. For example, it may be necessary to require accredited coaches or other support staff to keep up-to-date on drugs in sport initiatives, policies and procedures as part of their professional development to retain accreditation.

The second group was everyone else the athlete might trust to help them with their sporting careers. An example of how this might work comes from trading shares. Anecdotally, a colleague of the author's researches in this field, and attends conferences on how to predict shares going up or down. My colleague overheard a group of fairly influential researchers sharing stories about which stocks to trade, based on what someone's uncle had told them was a good purchase rather than their own mathematical models. This fable makes the important point that Kim and Jim may be more willing to trust the advice of their parents than the advice of the 'experts'. That is, the source of information may be less than optimal for making an informed decision about their use of performance enhancers.[36]

The experience of the mother of the emerging elite athlete was telling in terms of this group of people being largely forgotten in relation to drugs in sport. The main point arising from the discussion at this point was that one way of getting rhetoric to become reality was to consider how best to use the 'non-expert' people the athlete trusts to influence their decisions one way or the other. This suggests that the good work done in educating elite athletes needs to be extended to their entire formal (e.g. coaches, sports medicine etc.) and informal (e.g. parents, siblings and friends) members in the sportsnet supporting the athlete. At this point the task of education becomes rather large, since educating those who know someone involved in sport becomes educating everyone. An interesting research question becomes, how one educates entire populations about such things.

Some take home messages

This session was very important for reinforcing the notion of theory building from the ground up. Observations from the invited guests made the team pause to consider drugs in sport issues from a new perspective. Thanks to the invited guests the team was exposed to the way in which people experiencing drugs in sport as part of their everyday lives think about and look at the same issue. One take home message for the team was thinking about the application of our ideas. As noted above, research is only valuable if it is used. That is, the value of the research might be measured in terms of its effect on policy, changing behaviour of athletes, helping our understanding of the role of drugs in sport, or defining an idea as irrelevant to drugs in sport. The session therefore achieved its aim of helping the team understand drugs in sport from a different perspective.

Some comments on the second workshop

The high expectation and anticipation from the first workshop were met in the second with the fruits of some hard labour. The second workshop was characterized by a lot of time consolidating and refining our ideas. Ideas from the first workshop were built upon to evolve new ways of understanding of 'drugs in sport' derived from the Hypothetical.

Developing the agenda

This essay provides an introduction to the sorts of issues confronting the researcher attempting to come to grips with understanding the role of drugs in sport, either as an experienced researcher or new entrant to the field. What emerges from this process is an underscoring of the scope of research in which a social scientist can engage. There is a significant range of ideas for researchers to advocate for or against towards developing a robust debate about the role of drugs in sport. From a different perspective, this essay also identifies what happens when a group of social scientists from across the disciplines converge to apply their training to an issue. The result is both an exciting and daunting amount of information and ideas that can be used towards developing an agenda to guide research into drugs in sport using social science methods.

Notes

1 This point is made by Backhouse *et al.*, *Attitudes, Behaviours, Knowledge and Education – Drugs in Sport*, 110 and 119.
2 For a discussion of the many ways to see sport, see Section 1 of Morgan and Meier, *Philosophic Inquiry in Sport* for a sound in-depth account, Coakley, *Sports in Society*, or Cashmore, *Making Sense of Sport.*
3 Leonard, 'Doping in Elite Swimming: A Case Study of the Modern Era from 1970 Forward', offers insights into the organization and administration of swimming, especially in relation to doping.
4 O'Dea, 'Consumption of Nutritional Supplements Among Adolescents: Usage and Perceived Benefits', and Peters *et al.*, 'Beliefs and Social Norms about Ephedra Onset and Perceived Addiction among College Male and Female Athletes'.
5 Tested in Series 3 of the BBC production 'Body Hits'; see http://www.bbc.co.uk/bbcthree/tv/bodyhits/index.shtml.
6 The discussion paper released by the Victorian Government, *Towards a New Approach to Deterring Doping in Sport*, offers some insights into translating doping policies to apply to the non-elite context.
7 Houlihan, *Dying to Win*, 59.
8 Nixon, 'A Social Network Analysis of Influences on Athletes to Play with Pain and Injuries', refers to such networks as a 'sportsnet'. The BMA, *Drugs in Sport: The Pressure to Perform*, provides a sound overview of the issues around social network analysis of the athlete.
9 Leeds and von Allmen, *The Economics of Sport*, offer an account of sports as a multi-billion dollar entertainment industry.
10 For example, Byrne and Mazanov, 'Sources of Adolescent Stress, Smoking and the Use of Other Drugs', and Grekin, Sher and Wood, 'Personality and Substance Dependence Symptoms: Modelling Substance Specific Traits'.
11 Reilly, 'Alcohol, Anti-anxiety Drugs and Sport'.
12 Laure, 'Epidemiologic Approach of Doping in Sport', argues that developing a profile of coaches' doping preferences is an important part in the development of an epidemiology of doping in sport.
13 Armstrong and Reilly, 'Blood Boosting and Sport'.
14 Cashmore, *Making Sense of Sports*, 97, expands on this point suggesting two different-*genera*; from *Homo Faber*, or working man, for those who see sports as a job and *Homo Ludens*, or playing man, for those who participate for pleasure.
15 See Murphy and Waddington, 'Are Elite Athletes Exploited?', for more on this point.
16 See Byrne and Mazanov, 'Sources of Adolescent Stress, Smoking and the Use of Other Drugs'.
17 Hoberman, *Mortal Engines*, and Waddington, *Sport, Health and Drugs*, present accounts of the historic and modern involvement of drugs in cycling. Carstairs, 'The Wide World of Doping', 267, claims swimming is a drug resistant sport through its status as a sport without equipment, although no direct evidence is offered to validate the claim.
18 Brantigan, Brantigan and Joseph, 'Effect of Beta Blockade and Beta Stimulation on Stage Fright'.
19 Durkheim, *The Elementary Forms of Religious Life, and The Rules of Sociological Method.*
20 Waddington, *Sport, Health and Drugs*.
21 Even if drug use were permitted to achieve equality at least in terms of drugs the issue of economic inequality would remain.
22 For example, Eric 'the Eel' Moussambani from Equatorial Guinea had never swum in a 50m pool before the 2000 Olympics; ABC Online, http://www.abc.net.au/sport/content/200408/s1172243.htm.
23 Some examples of this literature are Tamburrini, 'Are Doping Sanctions Justified?'; Savulescu, Foddy and Clayton, 'Why We Should Allow Performance Enhancing Drugs in Sport'; and Schneider and Butcher, 'An Ethical Analysis of Drug Testing'. Miah, *Genetically Modified Athletes*, gives an in-depth account of the harm argument.
24 A point made by Mazanov, 'Managing Anti-doping in Sport: Public Past or Private Future?'
25 Verroken, 'Drug Use and Abuse in Sport'.
26 Foresight, 'Drugs Futures 2025', from www.foresight.gov.uk; and Mehlman, 'Cognition-enhancing Drugs'.
27 This line of argument is developed by Cashmore, *Making Sense of Sports.*
28 If a country has a zero tolerance policy that is applied equally in any sector, including sport, then sport has no special status. What creates the imbalance is that sportspeople are barred from using certain substances and methods that the rest of society may use freely. Further, players associations in Australia report fears their government would withdraw funding from minority sports to force them to take up zero tolerance illicit drugs policies, despite the BMA advocating for harm minimization approaches

(see Brett Harris and Stuart Honeysett, http://www.theaustralian.news.com.au/story/0,22396428-2722,00.html?from = public_rss).

29 Houlihan, *Dying to Win*, 145, expands on this point. For example, the Nazis were unable to change the rules of the International Olympic Movement to prevent Jesse Owen from competing; they had to submit to the rules of the sport in the attempt to demonstrate their political and ideological views.

30 For an accessible and expanded discussion of chaos theory from which this example comes, see Gleick, *Chaos: Making a New Science*.

31 Nixon, 'A Social Network Analysis of Influences on Athletes to Play with Pain and Injuries', and Murphy and Waddington, 'Are Elite Athletes Exploited?', for an expanded discussion on this point.

32 Strelan and Boeckmann, 'Why Drug Testing in Elite Sport does not Work', report using such scenarios with Australian professional athletes.

33 UK Sport, 2005 *Drug-Free Sport Survey*.

34 See the Victorian Government, *Towards a New Approach to Deterring Doping in Sport*. Girginov, 'Creating a Corporate Anti-doping Culture', also discusses WADA acting globally and acting locally.

35 The British Medical Association note this issue as a concern in, BMA, *Drugs in Sport: The Pressure to Perform*.

36 Laure and Binsinger, 'Adolescent Athletes and the Demand and Supply of Drugs', note that 69.7% of the adolescents surveyed trusted their PESM suppliers, mainly their friends, parents or family medical practitioner.

References

Armstrong, D.J., and T. Reilly. 'Blood Boosting and Sport'. In *Drugs in Sport*, 4th ed., edited by D.R. Mottram, 207–27. New York: Routledge, 2005.

Backhouse, S., J. McKenna, S. Robinson, and A. Atkin. *Attitudes, Behaviours, Knowledge and Education – Drugs in Sport: Past, Present and Future*. Montreal: WADA, 2007.

BMA. *Drugs in Sport: The Pressure to Perform*. London: BMJ Publishing Group, 2002.

Brantigan, C.O., T.A. Brantigan, and N. Joseph. 'Effect of Beta Blockade and Beta Stimulation on Stage Fright'. *The American Journal of Medicine* 72 (1982): 88–94.

Byrne, D.G., and J. Mazanov. 'Sources of Adolescent Stress, Smoking and the Use of Other Drugs'. *Stress Medicine* 15 (1999): 215–27.

Carstairs, C. 'The Wide World of Doping: Drug Scandals, Natural Bodies, and the Business of Sports Entertainment'. *Addiction Research and Theory* 11, no. 4 (2003): 263–81.

Cashmore, E. *Making Sense of Sports*, 4th ed. Abingdon: Routledge, 2005.

Coakley, J. *Sports in Society: Issues and Controversies*. Sydney: McGraw-Hill, 2007.

Durkheim, E. *The Elementary Forms of Religious Life*. New York: George Allen & Unwin Ltd, 1915.

Durkheim, E. *The Rules of Sociological Method*. London: Free Press, 1938.

Girginov, V. 'Creating a Corporate Anti-doping Culture: The Role of Bulgarian Sports Governing Bodies'. *Sport in Society* 9, no. 2 (2006): 252–68.

Gleick, J. *Chaos: Making a New Science*. New York: Penguin, 1988.

Grekin, E.R., K.J. Sher, and P.K. Wood. 'Personality and Substance Dependence Symptoms: Modelling Substance Specific Traits'. *Psychology of Addictive Behaviours* 20, no. 4 (2006): 415–24.

Hoberman, J.M. *Mortal Engines: The Science of Performance and the Dehumanisation of Sport*. New York: Free Press, 1992.

Houlihan, B. *Dying to Win*, 2nd ed. Strasbourg: Council of Europe Publishing, 2002.

Laure, P. 'Epidemiologic Approach of Doping in Sport'. *Journal of Sports Medicine and Fitness* 37 (1997): 218–24.

Laure, P., and C. Binsinger. 'Adolescent Athletes and the Demand and Supply of Drugs to Improve their Performance'. *Journal of Sports Science and Medicine* 4 (2005): 272–7.

Leeds, M.A., and P. von Allmen. *The Economics of Sports*, 3rd ed. Boston, MA: Pearson International, 2008.

Leonard, J. 'Doping in Elite Swimming: A Case Study of the Modern Era from 1970 Forward' In *Doping in Elite Sport: The Politics of Drugs in the Olympic Movement*, edited by W. Wilson and E. Derse, 225–39. Champaign, IL: Human Kinetics, 2001.

Mazanov, J. 'Managing Anti-doping in Sport: Public Past or Private Future?' Paper presented to Sporting Traditions XVI, Biennial Conference of the Australian Society for Sports History, Canberra, Australia, July 2007.

Mehlman, M.J. 'Cognition-enhancing Drugs'. *The Milbank Quarterly* 82, no. 3 (2004): 483.

Miah, A. *Genetically Modified Athletes: Biomedical Ethics, Gene Doping and Sport*. London: Routledge, 2004.

Morgan, W., and K. Meier. *Philosophic Inquiry in Sport*, 2nd ed. Champaign, IL: Human Kinetics, 1995.

Murphy, P., and I. Waddington. 'Are Elite Athletes Exploited?' *Sport in Society* 10, no. 2 (2007): 239–55.

Nixon, H.L. 'A Social Network Analysis of Influences on Athletes who Play with Pain and Injuries'. *Journal of Sport and Social Issues* 16, no. 2 (1992): 127–35.

O'Dea, J. 'Consumption of Nutritional Supplements Among Adolescents: Usage and Perceived Benefits'. *Health Education Research* 18, no. 1 (2003): 98–107.

Peters, R.J., L.F. Adams, J.B. Barnes, L.A. Hines, D.E. Jones, K.M.A. Krebs, and S.H. Kelder. 'Beliefs and Social Norms about Ephedra Onset and Perceived Addiction among College Male and Female Athletes'. *Substance Use and Misuse* 40 (2005): 125–35.

Reilly, T. 'Alcohol, Anti-anxiety Drugs and Sport'. In *Drugs in Sport*, 4th ed., edited by D.R. Mottram, 258–87. New York: Routledge, 2005.

Savulescu, J., B. Foddy, and M. Clayton. 'Why We Should Allow Performance Enhancing Drugs in Sport'. *British Journal of Sports Medicine* 38 (2004): 666–70.

Schneider, A., and R. Butcher. 'An Ethical Analysis of Drug Testing'. In *Doping in Elite Sport*, edited by W. Wilson and E. Derse, 129–52. Champaign, IL: Human Kinetics, 2001.

Strelan, P., and R.J. Boeckmann. 'Why Drug Testing in Elite Sport does not Work: Perceptual Deterrence Theory and the Role of Personal Moral Beliefs'. *Journal of Applied Social Psychology* 36 (2006): 2909–34.

Tamburrini, C. 'Are Doping Sanctions Justified? A Moral Relativistic View'. *Sport in Society* 9, no. 2 (2006): 199–211.

UK Sport. *2005 Drug-Free Sport Survey*. London: UK Sport, 2005.

Verroken, M. 'Drug Use and Abuse in Sport'. In *Drugs in Sport*, 4th ed., edited by D.R. Mottram, 29–63. New York: Routledge, 2005.

Victorian Government. *Towards a New Approach to Deterring Doping in Sport*. Melbourne: Sport and Recreation Victoria, 2006.

Waddington, I. *Sport, Health and Drugs: A Critical Sociological Perspective*. London: E & FN Spon, 2000.

Performance enhancement and drug control in sport: ethical considerations

Dennis Hemphill

School of Sport and Exercise Science, Victoria University, Melbourne, Australia

Performance enhancing drug use in sport is regarded as a crisis requiring comprehensive and often drastic measures to redress it. This essay examines critically the ethical foundations and implications of the major arguments that are mounted to oppose and control drug use in sport. Some of the most common arguments are based on appeals to naturalness, fairness, health and the spirit of sport. Others relate to the interplay of individual rights and community values, including those of sport. Not so common are the ethical issues that relate to the status of athletes as moral agents in high-tech sport and the ethical implications of 'zero tolerance' approaches to drug control. The essay concludes by identifying several avenues for further ethical scrutiny.

Introduction

It is quite clear that sport, whether it is at the local, national or international level, has embraced technology as a way of enhancing performance. Elite, amateur and even recreational athletes are benefiting increasingly from a number of recuperative and performance-enhancing technologies. These may range from physiological tests, surgical 'reconstructions', muscle fibre typing and biomechanical computer modelling, to psychological counselling, nutritional supplementation, as well as specialist coaching and state-of-the-art equipment and training facilities.

It is also quite clear that sport has shifted from a largely playful, amateur activity to a business-like professional enterprise. The emergence of sporting champions now appears to be less a matter of chance, 'gentlemanly' class privilege, or sheer personal determination, and more a matter of systematic state planning and corporate sponsorship. The large-scale economic and political interests served by gold medal and record breaking performances suggests that sport is fast becoming the competition between national systems or corporations with their respective stables of athletic performers.

At the same time, sport holds a special place in the public imagination. The use of performance enhancing means such as anabolic steroids, erythropoietin (EPO) and human growth hormone in sport is rife and, according to many, poses a threat to the integrity of sport. The menace of doping is thought to be so serious that it warrants global efforts to promote athlete education, comprehensive drug testing and stiff penalties for offenders. Sport philosophy, and sport ethics in particular, can shed some light on the interests and values at stake in our high-performance sport world.

How sport philosophy looks at drug control in sport

Sport philosophy is a discipline that critically assesses various truth, reality and value claims made about sport. With respect to the performance-enhancing drug issue, sport philosophy does all three. That is, it examines:

- the soundness of the arguments used to justify anti-drug policies and practices;
- it explores the nature and 'spirit' of sport that underpin doping control policy and practice; and,
- it helps to identify and sort out values (e.g. individual rights, community values) in sport, especially when they are inconsistent, ambiguous or simply clash.

Following Miah's discussion of science and the media, the ethicist's role should be 'pedagogic' and 'explain the range of moral concerns about a given case'.[1] Philosophers do this in order to promote more informed public opinion and policy on sport matters.

Before launching into the ethical considerations, it is first necessary to accept certain premises: drugs do indeed enhance performance and they can produce harmful side effects. This move is required so that empirical claims about the efficacy and/or harm produced by this class of performance enhancing agents do not sidetrack the discussion of the ethical issues. Also, the word 'drugs' will be used to include anabolic steroids, EPO and human growth hormone.

What sport philosophy has done

The case against drugs in sport

There are a number of conventional arguments used to support drug bans in sport. These include appeals to naturalness, fairness, health and harm to others.

Naturalness

On this traditional account, sport is thought to be the testing of natural abilities, that is, unaided by substances or methods external to the athlete. Performance enhancing drugs tamper with the body and interfere with nature. Thus, drugs should be banned because they introduce artificial, foreign substances into the body to help produce training or performance enhancements that could not be achieved otherwise.

Fairness

On the fairness account, it is argued that the use of drugs in sport should be banned because the use of a prohibited substance gives the user an unfair training and performance advantage over other athletes. One way of looking at this argument is to claim that athletes have a contractual obligation of sorts to abide by the rules governing a sport, and the use of a prohibited substance breaks a stated or implicit agreement. The effect of the rule violation is to change the conditions of play without the consent of other athletes, which can be considered unfair in its own right.

The more substantial effect of the rule violation is the unfair training or performance advantage it is thought to afford the rule-breaker. Fairness in sport is understood largely as the provision of a 'level playing field', that is, relatively balanced conditions of play in order to produce unpredictability of outcome – a desirable feature of sport. The rules stipulate the acceptable means to be used in the sport, and to gain an unfair advantage by intentionally using a prohibited means in training or in performance is considered to be cheating.

Health

On this view, drug prohibition is justified owing to the fact that the use of certain drugs or other performance-enhancing methods poses significant short- and/or long-term health hazards to athletes. Sport authorities, bolstered perhaps by a legal 'duty of care', may feel justified in banning certain practices, methods or substances that are considered dangerous or harmful in training or on the playing field. Young athletes, in particular, perhaps unaware of the effects of drugs, need to be protected from potentially harming themselves.

Harm to others

In addition to preventing self-harm, drug bans are often justified on the basis of the preventing harm to others. One such harm is coercion. An athlete using prohibited means can be thought to 'coerce' or force other athletes to employ similarly illicit and potentially dangerous means. The drug-clean athlete, for example, is put in the dubious position of having to consider cheating and enduring potential self-harm out of fear of being less competitive.

The harm to others argument is often extended to include the effect that adult drug use in sport can have on young athletes. Children are thought not to have the experience and maturity to make voluntary and informed choices with respect to drugs in sport. As a result, adult drug use in sport should be prohibited, as adult athletes are influential role models for impressionable young athletes.

How the case stacks up

The naturalness, health, fairness and harm to others arguments are some of the most common ones used to prop up anti-drug policy in sport. However, they are not without their problems; some that relate to clarity and others to consistency. The meaning of terms needs to be clear if they are to do the ethical work expected of them. As 'rational' human beings, we expect policies and rules to be applied even-handedly, with special cases requiring convincing explanations.

While the appeal to 'naturalness' is supposed to help draw the line between acceptable and unacceptable means of performance enhancement, the meaning of 'naturalness' is not entirely clear. If 'natural' means unaided by substances or methods external to the body, it is hard to imagine any aspect of life, let alone sport, that is natural. In sport, performance is routinely aided by training, dietary supplementation and a range of other substances or methods that can be considered 'artificial' and external to the athlete.[2] The inconsistency of this argument lies in singling out drugs for prohibition when there is a range of 'unnatural', yet acceptable, performance enhancers.

One of the problems with the health argument lies in the determination of what 'health' means with respect to the athletic population. It may be inappropriate to judge athletes by a standard of health thought to be more appropriate to a 'normal' population.[3] That is, athletes 'push the envelope', often risking life and limb in training and competition, as part and parcel of what it means to engage in an athletic way of life. There is also the problem of inconsistency here. While danger and risk is inherent in high performance sport, drugs are subject to distinctive exclusion.

The fairness argument is also thought to be inconsistent because there are many advantages that favour the performance prospects of some athletes over others, yet remain unquestioned.[4] Besides natural endowment, other more significant inequalities include the availability to some athletes of greater funding, as well as access to superior training/rehabilitation facilities, equipment, technology, coaching and other sport science or administration support. The inconsistency of the argument lies in the fact that, while so many other inequalities exist that can create unfair performance advantages for some athletes, drugs are singled out for special scrutiny and prohibition.

The weakness of the 'coercion' argument lies in the fact that it presupposes that the pressures to use drugs are somehow worthy of scrutiny and prohibition in ways that other competitive pressures are not.[5] It is not at all clear how drugs can be distinguished from other competitive pressures. If athletes choose especially difficult weight training or running programmes that carry with them certain risks, can it be said that these athletes are forcing others to engage in them? Left untouched are other equally dangerous or risky training regimens that can be seen to apply coercive pressure on other athletes.

The 'bad example to children' justification for drug control also falters. Restrictions exist to the freedom of adult athletes to use dangerous drugs to enhance performance or to use so-called recreational drugs that may sully the reputation of sport. Yet, restrictions do not exist on the freedom of adults in numerous other areas (e.g. arduous training programmes, alcohol consumption, poor diet) where they may also set a bad example to children.[6]

So, what is the solution here? The demonstration of consistency in the case of drugs in sport would require either universal prohibition or universal access. In the former case, there may be a number of unhealthy, dangerous and harmful practices, besides drugs, that would have to be eliminated in sport. In the latter case, any and all performance enhancers that might give one athlete an advantage over another would have to be made available to all athletes.[7] Both options would require costly efforts to either enforce wide-ranging prohibitions or to implement a global resource (e.g. facilities, equipment, scientific training and rehabilitation, specialist coaching) redistribution scheme to produce a level playing field. Alternatively, to avoid the charge of inconsistency, the onus is on sport authorities to demonstrate why drugs should be singled out for special scrutiny and prohibition when there are so many other performance enhancers that may be unnatural, unhealthy, unfair or cause harm to others.

In spite of these conceptual and logical problems, there still appears to be what Lavin calls 'pervasive disapproval' of drugs in sport.[8] This has prompted sport philosophers to continue seeking explanations as to why this is the case. There are a number of ethical perspectives, derived from criteria both external and internal to sport, that can provide some useful insights and guidance here. These include 'respect for persons' and an appeal to 'goods' that are internal to sport as a practice community.

Respect for persons

Implicit in some cases against drugs in sport is the view that their use undermines a principal feature of being human: personhood. Being a person is thought to be more than simply a machine-like thing that is acted upon or an object to be used as a means by someone else. Rather, an essential feature of personhood is thought to be self-determination. To be self-determining is to have the opportunity and ability to weigh up the pros and cons of alternative courses of action, make decisions without undue reliance on others, and accept responsibility for our choices.[9] In popular terms, personhood refers to the ability to 'stand on your own two feet', or 'be your own person'.

Related to this, at times, is the view that life's hardships should be met head-on and overcome through hard work, self-discipline and perseverance. Life's challenges and problems should not be avoided or made easier by the use of drugs, a view that Klerman refers to as 'pharmacological Calvinism'. It implies that drug use should be condemned because it is seen as a crutch or as a short cut that diminishes self-reliance, or as Klerman avers: honesty, sincerity and directness of response.[10]

These views have some currency in sport. While the outcome of a sport competition can be influenced by luck or injury, there is still a significant value attached by athletes and spectators to the link between success and self-determined effort. Victories or personal best performances resulting from sheer luck, or through opponent injury or default, are often deemed 'hollow'. Similarly, gross inequalities in skill level between opponents, which produce lop-sided outcomes, are often thought to take the gloss off victory.

For Simon, the ideal of competition is conceptualized as a mutually challenging quest for excellence between persons.[11] This means that competition involves the disclosing and testing of the skills and powers of an athlete in response to the valuable challenges served up by the opponent. As a test of persons, sport is thought to provide athletes with the opportunity to 'test their mettle' that is, demonstrate and extend their technical skills and personal discipline, courage, tactical ingenuity, perseverance and other characteristics of sporting prowess.

On these accounts, drug use can undermine what it means to be a person in sport. For Simon, the use of drugs changes sport from being a test of persons to be a test of the ability of the body to adapt to an external chemical agent.[12] That is, the use of drugs is seen to reduce the athlete's responsibility and credit for the performance. This, in turn, undermines the basis of respect amongst and for athletes. Richard Pound, chairman of the World Anti-Doping Agency (WADA), echoes this view when he states, 'Competitions should still be won through hard work, training and dedication'.[13] Thus, drug bans can be justified on the basis of upholding the value attached to personal effort, self-reliance and responsibility in sport.

Human freedom and paternalism

While drug bans can be justified on the basis of upholding personhood, the argument is not without its problems. It can be countered by the view that drugs, whether for recuperation or performance enhancement, actually provide an opportunity for athletes to work even harder at excelling in sport. That is, by speeding recovery from training or injury, drugs may permit athletes to train more frequently, for longer periods of time and with more intensity. So rather than diminishing personhood, drug use may actually increase personal effort and responsibility.

Furthermore, there are those who argue that doping is consistent with the nature of persons and the spirit of sport. Savulescu, Foddy and Clayton, for example, argue 'biological manipulation embodies the human spirit – the capacity to improve ourselves on the basis of reason and judgment'.[14] For Tamburrini, doping substances and techniques 'have everything to do with the essential purpose of the athletic contest: to expand the limits of our capacities'.[15] Shogan concurs with Konig that the constitutive demand of the sport discipline is to push towards human performance capacity.[16] Echoing Bronowski's celebration of the runner whose actions are 'an adventure in freedom' in order to explore the limits of one's strength, Brown encourages the use of innovative substances and techniques in sport that have the potential to expand self-knowledge.[17]

A further problem with the personhood argument has to do with the apparent contradiction between the value attached to self-determination and the power of sport authorities to deny an athlete's choice to use drugs. When we forbid individuals from doing something or impel them to act in some way on the grounds that we know what's in their best (health or personal) interests, this intervention is referred to as 'paternalism'.[18] It is defined by Dworkin as 'the interference of a state or a person with another person, against their will, and justified by a claim that the person interfered with will be better off or protected from harm'.[19]

Where it can be shown that a person lacks the capacity to make an informed or voluntary choice, interference may be justified. This is generally referred to as 'soft paternalism', and has special relevance in the case of children. Due to lack of training and experience, children often and inadvertently undertake dangerous activities and are not aware of the consequences of their actions. As a result, restrictions on individual liberty through banning drugs and other dangerous or unhealthy practices may be justified on the basis of preventing significant harm. In such cases it seems clear that paternalistic interference is not only permissible but may indeed be obligatory to prevent harm and allow for a full flourishing of the young athlete's potential.[20]

However, when paternalism is exercised over informed and consenting adults, this type of paternalism, referred to as 'hard' paternalism, is another matter. It is difficult to justify because it denies in adults the very feature of self-determination that we value and come to expect of them as 'persons'. On this account, 'if athletes prefer the gains that the use of drugs provide along with the possible side effects to the alternative of less risk but worse performance, external interference with their freedom of choice seems unwarranted'.[21] Thus, to justify drug prohibitions the onus is on the sport authorities to demonstrate that an athlete's choice to use performance-enhancing drugs was uninformed and involuntary, and/or that the consequences of such drug taking causes harm to others.

The notion of personhood has some normative force. However, when applied to the drug control issue, this largely individualistic notion of what it means to be a person renders two seemingly contradictory results. On the one hand, the appeal to self-determination makes the use of drugs appear as a prop that diminishes personal effort and responsibility. On the other hand, the appeal to self-determination suggests also that restricting the voluntary and informed choice of adult athletes when it comes to drug use is ethically questionable.

Sport as a practice community

To speak about sport as a practice community is to regard sport as a cooperative social activity that promotes the pursuit and achievement of goods internal to the activity.[22] Goods internal to a practice (e.g. research, teaching, medicine, ballet, football) refer to the purpose of the activity and the shared standards of technical, ethical or aesthetic excellence that guide its achievement. For Stout, these internal goods 'can be specified only in terms drawn from the activity itself, recognized only by people experienced in the activity and realized only by participating in the activity well as judged by its standards of excellence'.[23] Unlike external goods (e.g. fame and fortune), the internal goods are inclusive, for their achievement benefits the entire practice community.

On this account, winning at all costs, including the use of drugs is unacceptable. Winning in sport has value not simply because of the external rewards it can generate for champions, but because it stands for something: practice excellence.[24] For MacIntyre,

> whether we are painters or physicists or quarterbacks or indeed lovers of good painting or first-rate experiments or a well-thrown pass – that its good can only be achieved by subordinating ourselves to the best standard so far achieved, and that entails subordinating ourselves within the practice in our relationship to other practitioners.[25]

In other words, an individual's efforts to achieve or extend the standards of excellence are intelligible and legitimate only within the context of certain shared purposes and acceptable means in the sport practice community.

Besides undermining the standards of excellence in the practice community, drug use can have a number of other unsettling social effects. It can force 'drug-clean' athletes, for example, to justify their record-breaking performances to a suspicious public. It can compel athletes faithful to a previous ethos to withdraw from competition or lower their expectations of success. It can pressure drug-clean athletes to adopt means that may inflict self-harm. Rule violations change the conditions of play without consent. Taken together, drug use can undermine the significance attached to the spirit of sport and compromise the sport's ability to promote its internal goods.

There are at least two important implications of this notion of sport as a practice community for understanding sport. First, it defines the athlete as person in social terms. That is, it adds a social element to what would otherwise be simply an individualist notion of personhood. Second, it provides a concrete 'inside' starting place to look for normative criteria to judge the acceptability or unacceptability of the means used to achieve success in sport.

While standards of excellence and internal goods are sport specific, and may undergo historical shifts, they are thought to provide a framework for judging when an individual action is thought to be an acceptable one and when it is cheating or unsporting. The Fosbury Flop, for example, defied convention and revolutionized the sport of high jump. The infamous 'underarm bowl' incident in cricket, however, was judged by the practice community (i.e. players, coaches, spectators, journalists) to be 'just not cricket', and sport authorities were quick to outlaw the tactic for what was considered the good of the game. The trick is to determine where the line is drawn in order to say that the introduction of one performance-enhancing tactic or substance is good for the game and that another is cheating or unsporting.

Sentimentality and solidarity

The justification of drug bans in sport has been based upon appeals to what is considered natural, healthy and fair, or to seemingly universal features of being a person or the ideal of competition. The appeal to the internal goods of sport is thought to provide a set of more grounded criteria to judge the acceptability of performance-enhancing substances and methods, including drugs. However, to accept that 'standards of excellence and internal goods are sport specific, and may undergo historical shifts', is to render senseless notions that there is anything like 'the' nature of persons, 'the' spirit of sport, let alone a timeless ideal of competition. In other words, the social is thought to go all the way down when it comes to defining persons or sport and what is appropriate behaviour.

Accordingly, what we refer to as the nature of persons or the spirit of sport, and the normative claims that flow from them, can be seen as historically contingent and subject to change. These notions can be described less as timeless universals and more as an historically grounded, but no less powerful, set of collective sentiments about what sport is (or what it should be).[26] In other words, the nature of sport and behaviour appropriate to it may be more an entrenched or preferred image rather than the way sport is in-itself.

Depending on the social context different values or interests may come to influence the constitutive rules, how the formal rules are interpreted and enforced, or who may be legitimately called a player.[27] In the name of 'pure' sport, the amateur code, for example, had the effect of ruling out certain types of participants (e.g. working-class or professional athletes) and certain types of behaviours. Another type of collective sentiment can be said to be operating in contemporary sport. For Burke, the act of drug taking 'grates on the sensibilities of enough of the practice community, with strong enough voices, to make us affix the label evil or immoral to any athlete who takes drugs'.[28] When combined with popular notions such as 'sport is healthy', 'the level playing field', 'sport builds character', and the link between success and effort (e.g. 'giving 110%'), there may be still enough sentimental attachment to uphold the view that drugs are antithetical to sport.

The upshot of this view is that there is no one set of standards of excellence or internal goods that are definitive of sport. The moral force of drug prohibitions depends on the strength and duration of the collective sentiments or consensus of the sport practice community. Lavin argues that current drug bans do not capture a timeless ideal of sport; rather, the prohibitions represent a 'democratic attempt to enforce and perpetuate widely accepted ideals'.[29] For Brown, the concepts of normality, health and fairness are tied up with moral and social commitments: by implication, where the line is drawn between performance enhancers that are acceptable and those that are not will depend on where we want to draw it.[30]

Lavin suggests that a consensus on drug bans should invoke a pervasive opinion (e.g. amongst managers, players, spectators and governing bodies about an ideal of sport), evoke a visceral dislike of means that compromise the ideal (e.g. of athletic excellence), and be mindful of longstanding practices in the sport.[31] In a similar vein, Fairchild suggests that a sport community's 'abject' or abhorrent reaction to drug use is more than a response to cheating or to its effect on the practice ideal of excellence.[32] It also threatens the sport's constructed social order, one that supports athletes' identity and meaningful way of life.

The appeal to collective sentiments and democratic preferences can help account for how the sport practice community can accept some unnatural, unhealthy and unfair practices, as well as some ideals of sport, but reject others. For Lavin, it is not enough for one stakeholder group (e.g. players, organizing bodies, spectators) to claim a consensus on behalf of the entire practice community; otherwise, drug regulations will be seen as impositions. Lavin also warns that widespread disregard and criticism of anti-drug regulations are clear signs that there are shaky grounds to claim a consensus.[33]

What sport philosophy needs to know

The above discussion points out that, while there may be no universal foundations, there appears to be enough public sentiment to uphold the view that sport and drugs do not mix. At the same time, sport is thought to be facing a drug crisis, one that requires global efforts to promote athlete education, drug testing and stiff penalties. Sport philosophy needs to explore the nature of the 'crisis' and examine critically what social interests may be served or sacrificed by the efforts to ban drugs in sport. Following Burke's suggestions, sport philosophy needs to examine whose sensibilities are grated the most, and whose voices are stronger than others, when it comes to drug use and control in sport.

Culture of performance enhancement

Drug prevention and control programmes in sport focus largely on the individual athlete as the source of the problem and as the target of education, surveillance and control. As a result, sport authorities may overlook other contributing factors. An alternative way of looking at drug use and control is to examine the role that the institution of sport has for rewarding high performance and promoting a high-tech scientific culture of performance enhancement.

It is not difficult to understand the institutional pressures, expectations and enticements of elite, professional sport. Heinila refers to the process as the 'totalisation' of sport. It involves the following, roughly fleshed out, process. The 'spiral of competition' operating in sport sets in motion a rise in performance standards, professional commitment and expectations for compensation. In themselves they can be compatible with the internal goods of sporting practice communities. However, mass media and other commercial involvements in sport accentuate the monetary or publicity benefits of sporting success for players and all those involved in managing and sponsoring sport. As the commercial value of sporting success increases so too do the temptations for players, coaches and managers and sponsors to employ dubious means.[34]

However, the choice to use drugs may not pose a moral dilemma for many athletes. In order to understand how this could possibly be the case, Houlihan argues:

> There is already in existence a culture, professionally supported and promoted, that encourages the treatment of healthy athletes with drugs. Even if the 'drugs' are simply those which are legally available (in terms defined by both the state and the IOC), such as vitamins and food supplements, the athlete is already developing the expectations and patterns of behaviour that might initially parallel drug use, but which are to most athletes part of a common culture.[35]

In other words, athletes exist in a sporting culture where the expectations, norms and incentives to enhance performance are in place.

In order to understand how athlete expectations and behaviour might initially parallel drug use, but then change to include drug use, one can consider the early socialization of athletes. Roberts and Hemphill suggest the following:

> From their earliest involvement, athletes begin to internalise two very powerful messages of high performance sport: first, that success is equivalent to high performance; and second, that the achievement of high performance is at least in part a function of reliance on forces (i.e., persons, processes, objects) outside of oneself. When combined and repeatedly reinforced along the long road to elite performance, the two messages may not only produce an impenetrable shield against the condemnations of using drugs, they very well may predispose an athlete to employ them as merely one among the many external forces deemed necessary for success.[36]

In other words, the decision to use drugs may not be that radically different to the decision to use other, more conventional performance enhancers. When socialized into a culture that fosters trust and reliance on the expert knowledge and methods provided by coaches, physiologists, doctors, psychologists, nutritionists and a host of other sport science professionals, athletes may see drugs as consistent with the sporting culture of performance.

This raises a number of interesting issues towards which sport philosophers could turn their attention. For one, drug use may represent less a moral failure on the part of athletes and more of a culture shift within sport that normalizes drug use. Part of the culture shift may also be due to the high stakes involved, the level of state and corporate investment in sport, and the returns expected from it. Athletes must continually deliver record breaking or medal winning performances to justify continued corporate and state sponsorship. A performance-enhancement culture in sport doesn't simply make the athlete's choice to avoid the use of drugs increasingly difficult; rather, it may frame the choice to use drugs as a rational thing to do.

This calls into question the status of athletes as persons and moral agents. Athletes over-socialised into a culture of performance enhancement can make sport seem akin to a syndicate performance, with outcomes less attributable to individual effort and increasingly to a host of external performance-enhancing substances, methods and sport science and management personnel. As a result, it is questionable if and what type of self-determination and moral reasoning syndicate-athletes are capable of. For all we know, athletes may see the drug bans as strictly a compliance issue rather than a moral one. As a result, what we understand by a 'person' and a 'practice community', and the normative direction they can provide, may have to be reassessed in light of the tendency to see athletes as syndicate performers in state- and corporate-sponsored sport.

War on drugs

The campaign against drug use in sport is based largely on a zero tolerance model, one that combines heavy penalties with random testing and education programmes. Anti-drug education programmes presume that athletes will heed the health, safety and fairness messages against their use. When combined with penalties and stringent testing regimes, the campaign is expected to induce more athletes to just 'Say no to drugs'.

Prominent in the public rhetoric of drug control in sport are the 'doping' and 'war' metaphors.[37] Lakoff and Johnson state that the purpose of metaphor is 'to use one highly structured and clearly delineated concept to structure another'.[38] For example, the war on drugs in sport has become the war on doping. Calling someone a dope is short for calling them a stupid person ('dope is for dopes'). The word 'dope' is slang for illegal street drugs; being on dope carries with it the social stigma of being a 'user' or a 'druggie'. The arguments supporting bans on doping (e.g. health, fairness) have been shown to be inconsistent, but Dingelstad *et al.* comment that it is largely the social stigma associated with the use of dope in larger society that is effective in propping up the campaign against doping in sport.[39]

In the name of drug-free sport, authorities make frequent reference to 'getting tough', and 'expanding the arsenal of weapons', in order to 'combat' or 'fight' doping.[40] According to Lakoff, just wars are portrayed as having victims, heroes and villains.[41] WADA, for example, wages a war against the 'drug cheats' to protect sport for the 'clean', honest athletes. The use of the war metaphor in this way highlights the righteousness of the campaign, and justifies the firm resolve and forceful measures required for victory.

However, the persistent use of the war metaphor can produce a number of ethically dubious consequences when applied to drug control in sport. It raises the efforts against drugs in sport to the status of a war, encouraging the public to equate their seriousness. As a result, the public are also encouraged to accept, in a manner akin to a patriotic duty, the extreme measures, sacrifices and casualties that often accompany military campaigns. The current war on terrorism, for example, demonstrates the relative ease with which the case was made for the expansion of police powers and the suspension of certain human rights and legal protections (e.g. privacy, presumption of innocence, right to a defence) in the name of security.[42]

Scarry's study of the structure of war demonstrates how metaphors are used to hide or marginalize human pain, injury and suffering.[43] For example, it is described as 'collateral damage' or as the unavoidable 'costs' of waging war. In sport, the war on drugs raises a number of ethical issues. Some are related to privacy: athletes must submit to witnessed urine sample collection and year-round random drug testing, as well as report their whereabouts to drug testing authorities when travelling.[44]

Other issues relate to the fairness of drug testing. The policy of strict liability means that athletes are 'guilty until proven innocent' if found with drugs in their body, regardless of intent. Fairness is also at issue when sport authorities replace the legal precept of 'beyond reasonable doubt' with 'comfortable satisfaction', thus lowering the standard of evidence required to charge and convict athletes.[45] Burke illustrates in two high-profile cases (Jessica Foschi and Andrea Raducan) how unjust, but 'tough', decisions by sport authorities can be defended on the basis of being a deterrent to future doping.[46]

Moreover, it may be unjust to attribute so much of the blame to athletes when their performances are becoming more a syndicate effort amongst athletes, sport scientists and state/corporate managers and sponsors. In a view shared by Savulescu *et al.*, Tamburrini goes even further. He suggests that the worldwide standardization of doping sanctions allows for no gradations of guilt or to speak of diminished responsibility: a doped athlete from a poor country coerced into using drugs by a totalitarian government is treated the same as an doped athlete from a wealthy country who has access to a wide range of legal performance-enhancing substances, methods and other resources.[47]

The 'war on doping' campaign exposes the lengths to which sport authorities will go to not simply protect sport, but to protect one version of sport over others. So prominent is the 'war on doping' metaphor, it can make the very questioning of the anti-drug campaign tantamount to being unpatriotic. Houlihan argues that athletes are 'routinely relegated to the margins of debate' by sport authorities who (falsely) presume that athletes' interests correspond to that of sport governing bodies.[48] Moreover, the war can stifle debate on alternative strategies for drug control (e.g. harm minimization), suppress research on safe performance-enhancing drugs or reduce the autonomy of national or local sport institutions to develop policies that suit their particular traditions and conventions.[49]

For sport philosophers to investigate sport in this critical manner is not to be read necessarily as an endorsement of drug use in sport. Rather, it is to question the foundations of drug bans and the implications they have for understanding a range of human values in sport. It is also a call for open and informed public debate.

A research agenda for sport philosophy

The escalation of the war on drugs in sport raises a number of challenging issues and problems for understanding performance enhancement and drug control in sport. Some of the responses above only scratch the surface, and there is plenty of room to refine or extend these views. The solution for many of these issues and problems may require more collaboration amongst colleagues in sport philosophy, social science and sport law. For example, it would be fruitful to examine the attitudes of athletes, spectators and other members of the sport practice community to determine just what measure of public solidarity exists to support drug control in sport.

These issues and problems associated with performance-enhancing drug use and drug control provides a number of opportunities for further research in sport philosophy. Based on what has been discussed above, a research agenda for sport philosophy might include the following:

1. The important notion of creating a 'level playing field', and the disparities that exist across sporting nations in terms of resources for sport, could benefit from an examination of distributive justice. In addition, there have been a number of human rights issues raised by the 'war on drugs' in sport, issues that could be informed by a more thorough exploration and application of theories of procedural or other forms of justice.
2. While this essay focuses on the issue of performance enhancement in sport, many of the arguments for and against drug control spill over into the 'recreational' drug use issue in sport. Drug control in places of work or in sport practice communities may be one thing, but something different, and perhaps more ethically troublesome, when it extends into private life. Sport philosophers would do well to explore further the 'public-private' domain issue and its relation to 'recreational' drug use and control in sport.
3. Some voices have been shown to be dominant and others marginalized when it comes to describing the nature of persons, the spirit of sport, and the social interests served by drug policies and practices. It might also be worth taking a look at how the drug control issue would be described if it were taken out of a largely criminological discourse and lodged more in, say, a medical one. Moreover, it might also be useful for philosophers to explore the ethical assumptions and implications of a range of drug control approaches and programmes in the general community to see how they might add to the performance enhancement and drug control debate in sport.
4. Finally, the rapid growth of a state/corporate-sponsored, professional and scientific culture of performance raises a number of issues about ethics and drug control in sport. It invites philosophers to consider in more detail the impact of this development on the current understandings of personhood, communities and sport. Alternatively, it may prompt sport philosophers to explore the extent to which its ethical vocabularies expand or limit the understanding of sport, performance enhancement and drug control.

Notes

1 Miah, 'Genetics, Cyberspace and Bioethics: Why Not a Public Engagement with Ethics?', 142.

2 Brown, 'Ethics, Drugs and Sport'; Lavin, 'Sport and Drugs: Are the Current Bans Justified?'; Roberts and Hemphill, 'Banning Drugs in Sport: Ethical Inconsistencies'.

3 Brown, 'Ethics, Drugs and Sport'.

4 Brown, 'Ethics, Drugs and Sport'; Simon, 'Good Competition and Drug-Enhanced Performance'; Roberts and Hemphill, 'Banning Drugs in Sport: Ethical Inconsistencies'. See also Jim Parry, 'Ethics and Doping', http://www.blues.uab.es/olympic/studies/doping/parry.htm.
5 Roberts and Hemphill, 'Banning Drugs in Sport: Ethical Inconsistencies'; Simon, 'Good Competition and Drug-Enhanced Performance'; Tamburrini, 'What's Wrong with Doping?'
6 Roberts and Hemphill, 'Banning Drugs in Sport: Ethical Inconsistencies'; Simon, 'Good Competition and Drug-Enhanced Performance'; Tamburrini, 'What's Wrong with Doping?'
7 Brown, 'Ethics, Drugs and Sport'; Savulescu, Foddy and Clayton, 'Why We Should Allow Performance Enhancing Drugs in Sport'.
8 Lavin, 'Sport and Drugs: Are the Current Bans Justified?'
9 Downey and Telfer, *Respect for Persons*.
10 Cited in Neville, 'Drug Use, Abuse, and Dependence', 327.
11 Simon, 'Good Competition and Drug-Enhanced Performance'
12 Ibid. See also Simon, 'Response to Brown and Fraleigh'.
13 See Richard Pound, 'Taking the Lead'. http://www.wada-ama.org/rtecontent/document/Play_ True_01_2005_en.pdf
14 Savulescu, Foddy and Clayton, 'Why We Should Allow Performance Enhancing Drugs in Sport', 67.
15 Tamburrini, 'What's Wrong with Doping?', 203.
16 Shogan, *The Making of High-Performance Athletes: Discipline, Diversity and Ethics*, 77. See also Konig, 'Criticism of Doping: The Nihilistic Side of Technological Sport and the Antiquated View of Sport Ethics'.
17 Brown, 'Ethics, Drugs and Sport', 19, 22.
18 Jim Parry prefers and uses the gender neutral term 'parentalism' instead of 'paternalism'. See http://www.blues.uab.es/olympic/studies/doping/parry.htm.
19 See Gerald Dworkin, 'Paternalism'. In *The Stanford Encyclopedia of Philosophy* (Winter), ed. E.N. Zalta. http://plato.stanford.edu/archives/win2002/entries/paternalism/.
20 Brown, 'Paternalism, Drugs and the Nature of Sport', 215.
21 Simon, 'Good Competition and Drug-Enhanced Performance', 210.
22 MacIntyre, *After Virtue*, 187.
23 Stout, 'Liberal Society and the Language of Morals', 51.
24 Schneider and Butcher, 'Why Olympic Athletes Should Avoid the Use and Seek the Elimination of Performance-Enhancing Substances and Practices From the Olympic Games'; Schneider and Butcher, 'For the Love of the Game: A Philosophical Defense of Amateurism'.
25 MacIntyre, *After Virtue*, 191.
26 Burke, 'Drugs in Sport: Have They Practiced Too Hard? A Response to Schneider and Butcher'; Burke and Roberts, 'Drugs in Sport: An Issue of Morality or Sentimentality?'
27 See English, 'Sex Equality in Sport', where she discusses a 'masculine bias' built into the very structure of sport. See D'Agostino, 'The Ethos of Sport', to understand how social context influences how the formal rules are interpreted and enforced. See Brown, 'Ethics, Drugs and Sport', and Meier, 'Restless Sport', for discussion of who may be legitimately called a player.
28 Burke, 'Drugs in Sport: Have They Practiced Too Hard?', 48.
29 Lavin, 'Sport and Drugs: Are the Current Bans Justified?', 236.
30 Brown, 'Ethics, Drugs and Sport', 21.
31 Lavin, 'Sport and Drugs: Are the Current Bans Justified?', 237.
32 Fairchild, 'Sport Abjection: Steroids and the Uglification of the Athlete', 82.
33 Lavin, 'Sport and Drugs: Are the Current Bans Justified?'
34 Heinila, 'The Totalization Process in International Sport'.
35 Houlihan, *Dying to Win: Doping in Sport and the Development of Anti-Doping Policy*, 137.
36 Roberts and Hemphill, 'Banning Drugs in Sport: Ethical Inconsistencies', 5.
37 For example, see Mendoza, 'The War on Drugs in Sport: A Perspective from the Front Line'.
38 Lakoff and Johnson, *Metaphors We Live By*, 61.
39 Dingelstad *et al.*, 'The Social Construction of Drug Debates'; Burke and Roberts, in 'Drugs in Sport: An Issue of Morality or Sentimentality?', suggest that public revulsion of drug use in sport, at least in the case of female athletes, may be more a response to gender transgression than to cheating. For example, the potential effects of anabolic steroid use in women (e.g. large muscles, smaller breasts, facial hair and deep voice) threaten socially constructed norms of femininity.
40 In the nine paragraph 'Chairman's Message' on the World Anti-Doping Agency website, Richard Pound makes five references to the 'fight on doping', three references to being armed with new or more

'weapons to combat doping', four references to 'clean' sport, and single references to the 'level playing field' and 'health, fairness and equality'. See http://www.wada-ama.org/en/dynamic.ch2?pageCategory.id=237.

41 See George Lakoff, 'Metaphor and War, Again'. http://www.alternet.org/story/15414/.

42 For example, the anti-terrorism laws under what is known as the USA Patriot Act, an acronym for The Uniting and Strengthening America by Providing Appropriate Tools Required to Intercept and Obstruct Terrorism Act of 2001.

43 Scarry, *The Body in Pain: The Making and Unmaking of the World.*

44 Thompson, 'Privacy and Urinalysis Testing of Athletes'; Schneider, 'Privacy, Confidentiality and Human Rights in Sport'.

45 Morgan, 'Fair is Fair, Or is it?: A Moral Consideration of the Doping Wars in American Sport'.

46 See Burke, 'Drugs in Sport and Foucauldian Anxiety'.

47 Savulescu, Foddy and Clayton, 'Why We Should Allow Performance Enhancing Drugs in Sport'; Tamburrini, 'Are Doping Sanction Justified? A Moral Relativistic View', 207.

48 Houlihan, 'Civil Rights, Doping Control and the World Anti-doping Code', 421.

49 Dinglestad *et al.*, 'The Social Construction of Drug Debates'; Tamburrini, 'What's Wrong with Doping?'

References

Brown, William. 'Ethics, Drugs and Sport'. *Journal of the Philosophy of Sport* 8 (1980): 15–23.

Brown, William, 'Paternalism, Drugs and the Nature of Sport'. In *Philosophic Inquiry in Sport*, 2nd ed., edited by W.J. Morgan and K.V. Meier, 215–21. Champaign, IL: Human Kinetics, 1995.

Burke, Michael. 'Drugs in Sport: Have They Practiced Too Hard? A Response to Schneider and Butcher'. *Journal of the Philosophy of Sport* 24 (1997): 47–66.

Burke, Michael. 'Drugs in Sport and Foucauldian Anxiety'. *Bulletin of Sport and Culture* 24 (October 2005): 7–14.

Burke, Michael, and Terence Roberts. 'Drugs in Sport: An Issue of Morality or Sentimentality?' *Journal of the Philosophy of Sport* 24 (1997): 99–113.

D'Agostino, Fred. 'The Ethos of Sport'. In *Philosophic Inquiry in Sport*, 2nd ed., edited by W.J. Morgan and K.V. Meier, 42–49. Champaign, IL: Human Kinetics, 1995.

Dingelstad, D., R. Gosden, B. Martin, and N. Vakas. 'The Social Construction of Drug Debates'. *Social Science and Medicine* 43, no. 12 (1996): 1829–38.

Downey, R.S., and E. Telfer. *Respect for Persons*. London: George, Allen and Unwin Ltd., 1969.

English, Jane. 'Sex Equality in Sport'. In *Philosophic Inquiry in Sport*, 2nd ed., edited by W.J. Morgan and K.V. Meier, 284–92. Champaign, IL: Human Kinetics, 1995.

Fairchild, David. 'Sport Abjection: Steroids and the Uglification of the Athlete'. *Journal of the Philosophy of Sport* 16 (1989): 74–88.

Heinila, K. 'The Totalization Process in International Sport'. In *Sport and International Understanding*, edited by M. Ilmarinen, 20–30. Berlin: Springer-Verlag, 1984.

Houlihan, Barry. *Dying to Win: Doping in Sport and the Development of AntiDoping Policy*. Strasbourg: Council of Europe Publishing, 1999.

Houlihan, Barry. 'Civil Rights, Doping Control and the World Anti-doping Code'. *Sport in Society* 7, no. 3 (2004): 420–37.

Konig, E. 'Criticism of Doping: The Nihilistic Side of Technological Sport and the Anti-quated View of Sport Ethics'. *International Review for the Sociology of Sport* 30, no. 3/4 (1995): 247–61.

Lakoff, George, and M. Johnson. *Metaphors We Live By*. Chicago, IL: University of Chicago Press, 1980.

Lavin, Michael. 'Sport and Drugs: Are the Current Bans Justified?' In *Philosophic Inquiry in Sport*, 2nd ed., edited by W.J. Morgan and K.V. Meier, 232–38. Champaign, IL: Human Kinetics, 1995.

MacIntyre, Alisdair. *After Virtue*, 2nd ed. Notre Dame, IN: University of Notre Dame Press, 1984.

Meier, Klaus. 'Restless Sport'. Presidential Address: Philosophic Society for the Study of Sport. *Journal of the Philosophy of Sport* 12 (1985): 64–77.

Mendoza, J. 'The War on Drugs in Sport: A Perspective from the Front Line'. *Clinical Journal of Sports Medicine* 12 (2002): 254–8.

Miah, Andy. 'Genetics, Cyberspace and Bioethics: Why Not a Public Engagement with Ethics?' *Public Understanding of Science* 14 (2005): 409–21.

Morgan, William. 'Fair is Fair, Or is it?: A Moral Consideration of the Doping Wars in American Sport'. *Sport in Society* 9, no. 2 (2006): 177–98.

Neville, R. 'Drug Use, Abuse, and Dependence'. *Encyclopedia of Bioethics*, Vol. 1, edited by W. Reich, 326–34. New York: The Free Press, 1978.

Roberts, Terry, and Dennis Hemphill. 'Drugs in Sport: Ethical Inconsistencies'. Submission to Commonwealth Government of Australia Senate Inquiry into Drugs in Sport, 1988.

Savulescu, Julian, B. Foddy, and M. Clayton. 'Why We Should Allow Performance Enhancing Drugs in Sport'. *British Journal of Sports Medicine* 38 (2004): 666–70.

Scarry, Elaine. *The Body in Pain: The Making and Unmaking of the World*. New York: Oxford University Press, 1985.

Schneider, Angela. 'Privacy, Confidentiality and Human Rights in Sport'. *Sport in Society* 7, no. 3 (2004): 438–56.

Schneider, Angela, and Robert Butcher. 'For the Love of the Game: A Philosophical Defense of Amateurism'. *QUEST* 45, no. 4 (1993): 460–9.

Schneider, Angela, and Robert Butcher. 'Why Olympic Athletes Should Avoid the Use and Seek the Elimination of Performance-Enhancing Substances and Practices From the Olympic Games'. *Journal of the Philosophy of Sport* 20–21 (1993–94): 64–81.

Shogan, Debra. *The Making of High-Performance Athletes: Discipline, Diversity and Ethics*. Toronto: University of Toronto Press, 1999.

Simon, Robert. 'Response to Brown and Fraleigh'. *Journal of the Philosophy of Sport* 11 (1985): 30–2.

Simon, Robert. 'Good Competition and Drug-Enhanced Performance'. In *Philosophic Inquiry in Sport*, 2nd ed., edited by W.J. Morgan and K.V. Meier, 209–14. Champaign, IL: Human Kinetics, 1995.

Stout, Jeffrey. 'Liberal Society and the Language of Morals'. *Soundings* 69 (Spring 1986): 32–59.

Tamburrini, Claudio. 'What's Wrong with Doping?' In *The 'Hand of God'? Essays in the Philosophy of Sport,* Claudio Tamburrini, 34–49. Gothenberg: Acta Universitatis Gothoburgensis, 2000.

Tamburrini, Claudio. 'Are Doping Sanction Justified? A Moral Relativistic View'. *Sport in Society* 9, no. 2 (2006): 199–211.

Thompson, P. 'Privacy and Urinalysis Testing of Athletes'. In *Philosophic Inquiry in Sport*, 2nd ed., edited by W.J. Morgan and K.V. Meier, 253–56. Champaign, IL: Human Kinetics, 1995.

Towards a sociology of drugs in sport

James M. Connor

School of Business, UNSW@ADFA, Canberra, Australia

A sociologically informed analysis of drugs in sport requires the researcher to focus upon social forces. It is a continuing flaw of the literature that the individual is prioritized over wider social forces. In this essay I aim to provide a representative sketch of how the discipline questions and critiques social problems like drugs in sport. This includes arguing for a critical challenge to the mythologies of sport and drugs, and why and how sport and play are different, and exposing the role nationalism and ideology play in encouraging doping. I conclude by suggesting four avenues of research: amalgamating sport theory with drug theory, the concept of the networked athlete, prevalence rates and public perceptions of performance-enhancing drug use. This essay is by necessity broad and introductory – highlighting the challenge faced by sociologists to engage with the issue and demonstrate the social forces at work.

Introduction

An elite athlete bolts the door to his room in a publicly funded sports training institute. The day has consisted of a range of training sessions and techniques devised by his coach, bio-mechanical scientists and fitness trainers. His body was timed, tested and observed – all to ensure peak performance. He was subjected to psychological examination and taught mental strategies to 'enable' winning. A nutritionist crafted his diet to achieve a perfect balance of carbohydrates, vitamins and minerals. He took six different supplements to ensure that his body had every necessary nutrient. A media appearance was carefully supervised by his manager, media liaison and sponsor representatives. Two hours of his day was consumed by physiotherapists and masseurs. His travel itinerary even factors in high altitude training before each competition. Every activity has been geared to *enhancing* his performance so that he can *win*. Yet some enhancements are banned. The question that any sociologist is compelled to ask is 'Why are some methods and drugs banned and not others?' Moreover, what reasons and common understandings justify why only some are banned? But not content with such 'answers', sociologists seek to explore the issue of drugs and sport by placing the analysis firmly into the social realm and away from individualistic explanations. We consider history, theory and evidence, and address the competing explanations to seek out a better way to understand sport and drugs and drugs *in* sport.

Sociologists have investigated the use and abuse of drugs for a long time, with landmark work being done in the 1940s.[1] Conversely the critical attention paid to sports has occurred more recently (from the 1970s onwards)[2] and been subject to much theoretical critique.[3] Research that combines the two in any sustained theoretically and experimentally informed way is limited. If one was to employ a sports analogy, the current form of the team is patchy, unfocused and in need of some coaching. This is a failing on the part of sociologists as there is a very rich body of theory and experimental techniques that could be applied to sport *and* drugs. Further, it should be noted that sociologists have offered complex and nuanced explanations of sport that are well grounded in theory. However, there has been a failure to communicate these ideas and translate them for a wider audience.

The purpose of this essay is to sketch sociological approaches to drugs in sport. I start by explaining what sociologists do and why they can sometimes be perceived as being overly critical of society. This critical, questioning approach to the world allows sociologists to make some insightful comments upon sport in society by 'busting myths'. The first myth that I question is how and why sport has evolved from play to organized activity over the past 200 years. I then consider the profound impact the shift to professional, profit-driven sport has had. Sport is also intimately tied to nationalism and I explain how nation states have used sport and encouraged drug use to further national and ideological goals. The final myths that require questioning are the propositions that sport is healthy (it is not) and fair (far from it). This allows me to then point to four avenues of research required to further our understanding of sport: amalgamating sport theory with drug theory, the concept of the networked athlete, prevalence rates and public perception of performance-enhancing drug (PED) use. My overall aim, along with all good sociology, is to encourage us to challenge and improve the way we understand our world.

How sociologists see the world

Distilled to its essence, sociology seeks to question society. Sociologists do this by challenging the taken-for-granted assumptions (myths) that are made about how and why we live the way we do. We want to push through the boundaries, the edges, the beliefs in how things are and question them. A central assumption that underlies the discipline is the argument that the way we live is a social construction, which means that sociologists believe that, rather than the world existing as it does for any innate reason, it is human cultures, societies and values (to name just three components) that shape the way we perceive reality. The 'common sense' understandings of the world are not natural or bound up in objective fact, but socially mediated, or to return to the earlier point, the way we understand the world is socially constructed. This does not mean that things are not 'real' – we know that they are – but that how we make sense of them is a result of how we have come to perceive the world. As Newman argues:

> The social construction of reality is a process by which human-created ideas become so firmly accepted that to deny them is to deny common sense. Of course, some features of reality are grounded in physical evidence – fire is hot, sharp things hurt. But ... reality is often based not on hard evidence but on such forces as culture and language, people's definition of the situation, self-fulfilling prophecies, and faith and incorrigible propositions.[4]

It is the role of sociologists to question these forces through theory building and testing.

Another way of looking at how we question the world is to consider what one of the great American sociologists, C. Wright Mills, said about the discipline. The *sociological imagination*[5] is the term that Mills coined to encapsulate the questioning of society: 'the idea is to use a variety of viewpoints ... and in this way to let your mind become a moving prism catching light from as many angles as possible'.[6] It is by using this variety of viewpoints that sociologists question society. Sociology starts with the idea that we all have differing perspectives. However a key strategy of the sociologist is to take advantage of these views as a way of illuminating the issue under enquiry; which, in our case, is the vexed issue of drugs and sport.

The use of a range of views, or to be more technical, theories, is both the strongest and weakest aspect of sociological thought. Our theories allow us to develop coherent understandings and explanations of social phenomena; however, because we have a variety of ways of seeing, or 'catching the light', sociology features contradictory theories and explanations. What I endeavour to do in this essay is identify the key contributions that certain theoretical perspectives offer for an understanding of sport and drugs. I also indicate the weaknesses in some approaches and indicate what further research needs to be carried out to further explicate drugs and sport from a sociological perspective. This is by no means an exhaustive review of the literature; the purpose of this essay is to canvass the general approaches and understanding that sociology has of drugs and sport.

An analytic framework

To explain an issue like the use of performance enhancing drugs (PEDs) in sport, C. Wright Mills would ask a sociologist to do four things:

1. consider the personal issues or troubles that concern people in society;
2. connect this to social issues, problems and forces;
3. place the issue in its historical context;
4. apply sociological theories, models and understandings to illuminate the issue.[7]

To start with Mills' first point, the use of PEDs in sport is a personal issue or trouble that concerns people. Critically, it is not an issue that merely affects a lone individual, but it is an issue that concerns many. Thus, while the need for the athlete to win and their potential use of drugs is a private affair, it has become a public issue because the use of PEDs has been banned. (For a deeper discussion on the relationship between private actors and public interest, see Houlihan.[8]) This is the connection between the acts of the lone athlete and the wider concerns of society. There are other connections between the individual athlete and society in this respect also – if the athlete is competing for a team or a country they are wrapped in a social *milieu*, although still an individual.

To continue utilizing Mills' approach, the sociologist then needs to consider the wider social forces, problems and issues that are part of drugs in sport. Thus, we would consider issues such as capitalism, the gendered nature of sport, the importance of national pride and the overriding need to win. The question that arises from this is how these issues impact on the decision of the individual athlete in relation to the use of PEDs.

The historical context is particularly important as it helps explain where we have been and how we got to the point we are now at. In terms of PEDs in sport, this means considering the origins of competitive sport and the development of the relationship between sport and society. It also entails considering the historical move from drug permission to drug prohibition and how the anti-drugs message in wider society has been replicated within sports.

Finally, to complete Mills' approach, a sociologist would seek to apply theories and models to understand the processes highlighted above; but more of these later.

The key assumption that has underpinned my discussion thus far is the sociological view that the individual is second to the social. That is, individualistic explanations of drug use in sport not only hide the real reasons for use but also continue to feed the view that sport is about the athlete alone. Sociologists reject any view that fails to acknowledge how the athlete is constituted in and by the society of which they are part. As Armour, Jones and Kerry point out, 'a social being cannot escape society in order to participate in sport, rather, society consists of structures and agents who constitute – and reconstitute – sport'.[9] What this means is that to understand drugs in sport one cannot examine the athlete-user alone; one must also seek to explain the social reality around sport. This broad approach of sociologists to examining the social context rather than merely the actions of individuals is very long in its tradition, and perhaps best summed up by a founder of sociology, Karl Marx, in 1852:

> Men make their own history, but they do not make it just as they please; they do not make it under circumstances chosen by themselves, but under circumstances directly encountered, given and

> transmitted from the past. The tradition of all dead generations weighs like a nightmare on the brain of the living.[10]

Marx's prosaic style aside, what his argument means for an issue like drugs in sport is that the decision of an individual athlete is not made alone, but within a set of circumstances already created for them. Those circumstances are of course part of the society that we inhabit.

To summarize the sociological approach to studying drugs in sport: sociologists argue that one cannot just focus on the actions of the individual athlete as these acts are made under the influence of a host of social forces and processes. As Armour *et al.* posit, the 'purpose of sports sociology is clear: it must study the sports/exercise person (at whatever level) as a social being in a particular social context; it must study social structures which endure and which have influence'.[11] It is the study of social forces that is the particular strength of sociologists.

What sociology has done

To understand the use of drugs in sport we first need to turn our attention to the question of just what sport is and how is it used, portrayed and played in society. In line with the sociological mission of questioning taken-for-granted assumptions about the world, this section critiques sport and assume that how it 'appears' may not be how it really 'is'. Firstly, I explore the concept of 'sport' and what sociologists argue to be the origins of sport. I then examine the explanations of sport that have informed most studies, including the few that enquire into drugs and sport. The aim is to approach the examination of sport from the perspectives around the broad categories of capitalism, masculinity, nationalism and hegemony. By following this line of explanation, I hope to provide some clarification of these perspectives as we tour what has already been argued.

Before exploring the origins of sport it must be noted that sport is part of, and cannot be separated from society, much like the individual. To view it as different is to imbue it with a particular character that sport does not possess, as Frey and Eitzen point out:

> to view sport as separate or different in this way may be problematic in light of the important part sport plays in our society. Sport is played at school, it dominates the media, it takes up our leisure time, sporting metaphors dominate our language and sports contests provide vehicles for the exhibition of national pride.[12]

Thus, I begin by placing sport in society (i.e. in its social context) and explore why sociologists claim that sport today is different from the physical games that preceded it.

Historic *play*; modern *sport*

Modern sport is just that, *modern*. Horne argues that it is 'a *modernist* creation of the late 19th century, as opposed to the considerable number of physical game contests and play forms that have existed throughout the world over several centuries'.[13] Miller, Lawrence, McKay and Rowe support this contention when they claim that 'sport of a regular and organized kind is the product of a social institution with its origins in Victorian England'.[14] Obviously we have had 'sporting' contests for much of human history, the ancient Olympics being a prime example of the durability of sporting challenges in society. The case these authors are making is that the way we play, watch and engage with sport is significantly different today. This difference is a result of sport becoming 'mixed up with the development of industrialism and capitalism, the spread of liberal democracy and the growth of mass communications'.[15] What this means is that sport is not something that is 'natural' human behaviour. The sporting contests we have today are a product of the forces that Horne identified, or, to phrase it differently, modern sport is played the way it is today because of the changes that have occurred in how we manage, produce and consume in our society. Thus, sociology challenges the assumption (or myth) that sport is 'natural' or 'normal'. It is a cultural activity with a social context.

This shift in how we perceive physical activity, from play to sport, is central to understanding how and why sociologists claim that sport today is different. Frey and Eitzen make the distinction about a transformation from play, which is playful activity for its own sake (*ludic*), to sport, which has an intrinsic purpose.[16] They define play as being viewed:

> as an activity where entry and exit are free and voluntary, rules are emergent and temporary, fantasy is permitted, utility of action is irrelevant, and the result is uncertain. Play has no formal history nor organization; motivation and satisfaction are intrinsic; and the outcome does not have serious impact beyond the context of the activity.[17]

Thus, play is profoundly different from the modern sporting contests we see and engage in. Just consider the focus on the scoreboard in modern sporting contests. Frey and Eitzen succinctly emphasize this point when they argue that modern

> sport is hardly voluntary; rules are formal, generalizable, and enforced by formal regulatory bodies; the outcome is serious for individuals and organizations not actually participating in the physical activity, and winning (the outcome) is more important than participation (the process).[18]

The emergence of sport is part of the broader changes in society that processes of modernity have wrought (roughly starting from the eighteenth century). The changes can be summarized by considering how sport has become an activity beyond just exercise and has become a serious industry itself.

Industrial sport; sport as profit

Sport as an industry is significant on the global scale, including the sports themselves, sporting-goods manufacturers, sports marketing, sports tourism, sports apparel, sports drinks, sports gambling and, of course, sports media. Estimating the global value of this is mind-boggling. Using just two examples (Australia and England) demonstrates how much money is involved. In Australia, in 2001, the Australian Bureau of Statistics reported that sports generated A$8.5 billion in income.[19] In the 2001 census 1% (83,008) of the workforce was engaged in sport and physical recreation.[20] In England, it was estimated that, in 2000, sport value-added GB£9.8 billion and employed around 400,000 people, just under 2% of the workforce.[21] It is undeniable that sport has become a global industry generating significant revenue.[22] However, what is curious about sport is that it is a unique industry, as Horne argues:

> where else would consumers (football fans) maintain high levels of consumption even if quality (success) declines and price rises? Indeed, continuing consumption (support) in the face of lack of success is seen as a true sign of commitment. Likewise, otherwise rational entrepreneurs will invest vast sums of money into commercial teams in pursuit of sports success without serious expectation of financial return ... Sport is clearly much more than simply another industry.[23]

Sport is more than just a money-making endeavour, as will be discussed shortly, but one cannot discount the importance of money in sport. It is a common argument of sociologists that sport has been, and is being, increasingly commercialized.[24] This commercialization of sport means that profit becomes the overriding motivation, eclipsing ideals of fair play and sport for the sake of sport (though lip service is paid to these ideals). As Frey and Eitzen argue: 'we should not be surprised that high-level sport has been transformed into a commercialized, commodified, and massified phenomenon'.[25] The reason, simply, is that there is profit to be made in sport.

The profit motive: athletes

The profit motivation, as a result of the professionalization of sport and involvement of the media in sport, means that there is now a single, all-powerful motivator in sport – *winning*. Victory has become the ultimate goal of sporting clubs, coaches and athletes and the rewards for winning are considerable.[26] Clubs and sporting bodies rely on payments by media interests for the broadcasting rights to their sport along with endorsements and sponsorship deals.[27] The key determining factor with respect to the saleability of these rights and securing of endorsements is the ability to win, or the possibility of it, which will, in the language of current media parlance, 'sell' the sport to the consumer. Athletes themselves must win or they will not get the contracts, sponsorship or government support that will enable them to continue winning. For the miniscule minority of sports people who do 'win' the rewards can be astronomical. The overriding need to win is summed up neatly by one of Nike's slogans during the 1996 Atlanta Olympics – 'Second place is the first loser'.

The desire to win, and thus, by proxy, to achieve financial and other, less tangible, rewards, can override moral restrictions that might otherwise prevent a person engaging in dubious activities. Winning in sport is a zero-sum structure: if I win you must lose.[28] This results in winning being the most important motivation, and, as Jones and McNamee argue, in sport

> the goal is not to equalize relations. The competitive principle in sport is precisely to secure victory (within the rules) which necessarily precludes the opponents from doing the same ... Any kind of physical or mental advantage is pressed in order to secure victory.[29]

If performance-enhancing drugs or methods can give one the competitive edge, with such rewards at stake, then it is not surprising that athletes will use them. I am not denying that there is still some reward in the 'sport for the sake of sport' position, but as Frey and Eitzen argue:

> their significance [intrinsic rewards] seems to be devalued by the rising importance of monetary rewards (legal and illegal) for athletes, the exaggerated importance of winning that translates into treating athletes as interchangeable parts, the increase in the incidence of athletes using performance enhancing drugs, and the association of athletic success with outcome goals of profit, visibility, entertainment, and community/organization prestige.[30]

If sport is a modern industry with profit being a driving force, then it is inevitable that PEDs will be used in sport. This is the case as generating profit relies on selling sport – the product – to consumers. Sociologists have argued convincingly that increasing commercialization and commodification of sport has fundamentally changed sport.[31] In the context of Australian sport we can see this with the professionalization of the major football codes and cricket. This process began in the 1970s and has advanced swiftly since.[32] The rise of Twenty/20 cricket and the Super 14 Rugby Union are prime examples as these two innovations are designed for consumer, media-driven consumption, and therefore to make money. In the case of Super 14 (previously 12) it was invented to drive pay-television subscriptions, and Twenty/20 is set to become an advertising and gate attendance bonanza as a quickened and supposedly more exciting form of cricket. In this respect Twenty/20 follows from the World Series Cricket innovation introduced by Kerry Packer in the 1970s primarily as a way of driving television audiences for cricket.

This change in sport has resulted in two groups making considerably more money from sporting endeavours – the owners and administrators of codes and teams – as well as a small minority of elite sportspeople. Continuing with the example from Australian cricket, Stoddart explains that in 1975 Australian Cricketers would receive about $2,000 each, plus minimal expenses, to tour England, while in 1984 they could earn up to $40,000 a season.[33] By 2004 the captain of the Australian Cricket Team earned $2.24 million.[34] This astounding increase in earnings for cricket is mirrored in all other sports. For example, elite professional football (soccer) players whose weekly income in the English League was capped at £20 in the 1960s can now earn £20,000 – a 1,000 fold increase.[35] While a case could be made that athletes have been very poorly rewarded in the past, the huge and growing financial rewards offered to the minority of successful athletes operates as a very powerful motivational force on all athletes, which can have only one impact on PED use.[36]

However, this focus on the few successful athletes (both in terms of money and success) obscures the legion of athletes who do not make it to the elite level. In reality, very few athletes will make it to the pinnacle of their sport and receive large monetary pay-offs. The half-life of top Australian Football League (AFL) players is three years, as highlighted by Riewoldt (a St Kilda player) who addressed draft inductees in 2005:

> To make the point, the [AFL players] association enlisted the help of St Kilda's young star Nick Riewoldt to address the class of 2005 at this year's draftee induction camp, held last month. Riewoldt, who entered the league in 2001, could not have been blunter. 'Take a look around', he said to the latest batch of AFL hopefuls. 'More than half the players here won't be in the AFL in three years' time. Not long ago, I sat in the same place as you and now more than half of those blokes have one [an injury].'[37]

The pressure on young hopefuls with such a short playing life can only encourage the use of anything that might give them an advantage and lengthen their career. Staying with AFL, most players have made a long-term commitment in trying to get into the senior ranks. This often involves sacrificing other career opportunities, education and life experience. The AFL Pathways programme is a system designed to train young players and eventually lead them into the AFL proper,[38] however, according to former players, 93% of players in the Pathway programme will never make it.[39] The key sociological point here is that the individual athlete in sport is expendable. There is a line of athletes ready to take their place at the top. This sort of pressure must encourage athletes to at least consider PEDs as a way of moving from being one of the 93% in the AFL pathway programme to one of only 7% playing top level Australian Rules.

The profit motive: institutions

The owners and administrators of sporting competitions, as the second key stakeholder, have a vested interest in maintaining the marketability of their sport to secure some of the increasing sponsorship and rights deals being offered. The English Premier League will earn GB£1.7 billion for the broadcasting rights of three seasons from 2007, compared with GB£1.02 billion for the previous three years.[40] The wealth and income generation of sport as an industry cannot be denied. This means sporting codes need to maintain as marketable a product as possible with which to compete. On one hand this does offer an incentive to reduce PED use, as scandals may be seen to diminish the value of the sport. However, practical experience would suggest that scandals, while damaging in the short term, have no long term impact. For example, the Olympics (winter and summer), Tour de France and professional baseball in the United States have all had serious PED scandals yet continue to attract sponsorship, broadcasting and, crucially, fan support.[41] Thus, as an administrator or team owner I might ask whether it is in my interests to ensure the best sporting spectacle that I can, and if this means enhancing performance, or turning a blind eye to the use of PEDs, then perhaps I will be tempted.

The Olympics has been converted from a celebration of amateur sporting success to a multi-billion dollar global brand. This has had a profound effect on the way sport is governed and how rules for drug use are created, tested and enforced. The influx of money has led to evidence of corruption, graft and greed within the IOC.[42] As Miller *et al.* argue: 'it is a sorry tale of greed and corruption' by the IOC.[43] The question that must be asked by sociologists then is how can an international body (the IOC) with no regulation by nation states be allowed to create and enforce a drug testing regime? It is akin to the foxes being placed in charge of the hen house. We must even question if the IOC, as embodied by WADA, is fit to oversee anti-doping.[44] Simply put, from a sociological point of view, there is far too much money at stake for bodies like the IOC to ever effectively and fairly enforce bans on PEDs. It is not in their interests to have continuing scandals plaguing sport, which is what the likely result would be if there was a proper system of enforcement. Further, the Olympics (like all sport) need records and milestones to be broken, as they make the sport more marketable and thus profitable. Given that there are undoubtedly a number of records set by athletes utilizing drugs, including many in track and field which have stood since the height of drug use amongst Eastern Bloc countries during the 1980s, without drugs the number of Olympic records broken would decline each games.[45]

Consequences of the profit motive

The source of this large increase in money in sport is primarily advertising. Marketers know that sport is a wonderful vehicle with which to contact consumers, especially harder-to-reach men under 35. This profit motive neatly leads us back to where we began this section, namely, that sport is now a commodified, commercialized form of entertainment that is sold to consumers. This argument about sport, if correct, leads us as sport sociologists to a number of profound conclusions. Firstly, while capitalism (and the profit motive) is the driving force behind sport it is *inevitable* that PEDs will be used by athletes and encouraged by coaches, administrators and owners. As Hemphill points out, 'as the commercial value of sporting success increases so too are the temptations for players, coaches and promoters to employ dubious means'.[46] This is because the overriding need for victory, for winning, for overcoming the other, is a central tenet of both sport and capitalism. The two very conveniently mesh. Secondly, athletes will be strongly encouraged by two aspects of the reward/punishment system inherent in capitalism. They will be pressured to use PEDs because the rewards on offer for winning the gold, coming first or being the 'best of the best' will outweigh any possible sanction that could be applied. Athletes will also know from long years of competition that there is a reserve army of others waiting behind them, and it does not matter to the public which athlete becomes the next world record holder, just that one does. This means that as an individual one is interchangeable and unnecessary for sport.

Sport is the nation; nationalised sport

Nation States have a long history of using sport as politics by another means. The twentieth century is marked by this particular combination, be it Hitler's Nazi Regime glorifying Aryans at the 1936 Berlin Olympics or the boycotts of the 1980 Moscow and 1984 Los Angeles Olympics.[47] Norbert Elias, a classical sociologist, made this very point as long ago as 1939 when he argued that, 'the competitive bodily exertions of people in the highly regulated form that we call "sport" have come to serve as symbolic representations of a non-violent, non-military form of competition between states'.[48] Sport is a central aspect of nation building and prestige creation.[49] The Australian Institute of Sport (AIS) is a prime example of the role the state plays in propagating sport for national identity. The AIS was set up partly in response to Australia's medal haul in the 1976 Montreal Olympics (one silver and four bronze medals), which was acknowledged as a poor showing for a supposedly sports-driven country like Australia.[50] Hogan and Norton estimate that each Olympic gold medal won between 1980 and 1996 cost the Australian taxpayer $37 million.[51] The significance of this government involvement is that the purpose of sport is not for the joy of physical activity (as articulated in the 'Spirit of Sport' statement of the WADC), it is about competition between nations and, at times, competition between competing political ideologies (fascism, communism and capitalism).

The involvement of governments in sporting endeavours leads to sport becoming a means to an end, be it prestige, wealth or national pride.[52] Sociologists question the use of sport to encourage nationalism because of the social problems this can lead to. As Hughson, Inglis and Free point out, 'mass media has repeatedly whipped up nationalist enmity amongst sport fans'.[53] The problem with nationalism is that it encourages an 'us *versus* them' attitude which, at its worst, leads to violence (witness football hooliganism), racism, war and genocide.[54]

Governments have also had a long history of encouraging the use of performance-enhancing drugs and methods so that their country can be successful.[55] The East German Communist Government is renowned for doping their athletes in the 1970s and 1980s.[56] More recently there has been continuing questions regarding Chinese athletes and claims of systematic, government-supported doping.[57] The significant point is that when sporting success is tied to national success there is always a risk of governments becoming involved in performance enhancing, both legal (training institutes) and illegal (doping). This offers further evidence that drug testing and punishment regimes focused on the individual are not going to prevent PED use when a government supports the use.

Healthy sport; fair play

The mythology of sport implies that sport is healthy and natural, something that is inherently good for the body and very often the soul. UNESCO proclaims that:

> Physical education and sport form an important part of educational systems and are key contributors to social, human and intellectual development. Both public authorities and private sector are thus united in their efforts to stimulate the general interest in sport and physical education, as they are clearly a powerful influence in:
>
> - promoting human values, fair play, ethics, well-being and healthy-lifestyle;
> - bringing together persons from different social, cultural and geographic background regardless of religion and ideology;
> - contributing to peace and human development.[58]

This view of sport, as somehow inherently a moral good, is a particularly virulent myth. Hargreaves points out that the common sense view of sport is 'that sport helps individuals to develop stable personalities and contributes to their well-being and all-round development, thus functioning to benefit society as a whole'.[59] However, sociologists argue quite convincingly that sport is neither healthy nor inherently moral.[60] Consider this picture of training:

> Athletes subject their bodies to inordinate levels of pain and injury and often over-train in distinctly unhealthy ways. Moreover, in the quest to improve performance, elite athletes from virtually all countries engage in blood doping; consume diuretics, hormones, steroids and stimulants; adhere to ascetic dietary regimes; and use aquadynamic and aerodynamic clothing and equipment. Many high level athletes train in national sports institutes that simulate climates and altitudes, elevating red-blood-cell counts. The Australian Institute of Sport even has a special facility known as Altitude House, where athletes sleep in chambers that stimulate a high-altitude atmosphere. Far from being 'natural,' elite sporting bodies are akin to docile cyborgs.[61]

The authors are making a very strong argument that sport is not a healthy activity, nor a fair, moral or natural one. Doping control agencies claim that health of the athlete is a key reason why drugs in sport need to be banned, with athlete health being one of the three criteria used to determine if a substance or method should be banned.[62] However, if the health of athletes is a concern then drugs are a miniscule part of their health 'problems'. To actually make elite sport healthy we do not need anti-doping codes, we need anti-training codes limiting the type and amount of training an athlete can do. We also need anti-competition codes restricting the number of games/meets/competitions in which an athlete can engage. Further, taking this argument to its conclusion means that any sport with a high risk of injury (in effect any contact or near contact sports; all football codes for example) should be banned.[63]

Perhaps even more telling in this debate is the sociological idea that 'health' itself is a social construction: there is no accepted definition of 'health'.[64] This argument asks us to consider how we discern between drugs for enhancement (i.e. doping) and drugs for recuperation? What sociologists have consistently and persuasively argued is that the health discourse of 'drugs being bad' is a socially constructed argument used to further the interests of particular interest groups in society and that there is no logical basis to the claim that sport is healthy (it is not) and that drugs are bad – it is too complex an issue for such a simplistic response.[65]

Medicalisation of sport

A sociological discussion of health and sport would not be complete without highlighting the concept of medicalisation.[66] The term medicalisation is used 'to explain the way in which the apparently scientific knowledge of medicine is applied to a range of behaviours that are not self-evidently biological, or even medical, but over which medicine has control'.[67] Medicine is gaining increasing control over aspects of our existence that it previously had no control over (for instance, child birth is often cited by feminist-inspired sociologists). In the realm of sport a physiotherapist, nutritionist and doctor have become fixtures in any elite team. This was not always the case; for example the Australian cricket team's renowned physiotherapist, Errol Alcott, first joined the team in 1984.[68] This process is important because it points to how and why medical doctors (the Madrid cycling investigation) and medical researchers (BALCO) have become involved in doping scandals. This is because medicine has become a key component of sporting success, thus it is inevitable that the practitioners are drawn into the culture of winning at all costs.

The myth of fairness

The last myth of sport that sociologists debunk is the idea of fairness. Sport is not remotely a 'fair' social activity and claims that it is the epitome of egalitarian, open and level competition are patently false. Sport is not fair at the outset because sport mirrors wider social inequalities, both at the individual and global level. For the individual, gender, ethnicity, class and spatial location (to name just a few dimensions of inequality) will determine a person's chance of being a successful athlete.[69] At a global level there is a simple reason why African athletes perform well at track events, but not field events or swimming – it is because running requires very little in the way of material resources. Conversely, a single Olympic-quality pole for pole vaulting costs at least US$500 (typically a vaulter would have a dozen poles and they break or wear out quickly), to say nothing of the bar, uprights, pit, bags and run up track. Similarly, the capital investment and maintenance cost of an Olympic standard 50-metre pool is beyond the means of many countries. Rich, developed countries can support athletes with institutes, scholarships, training support, facilities and equipment.

These cross-national differences are mirrored for the individual as well. If we start with gender, you are likely to be more successful and better rewarded if you are a male athlete. It is a truism that male sport is favoured over female sport. Further, there are still sports where women are excluded on the basis of their sex (for example, boxing only started allowing women in the ring in the closing stages of the twentieth century). Part of this can be explained by acknowledging the dominance of patriarchal societies which systematically favour men over women. Even when women's sport receives media coverage it is often sexualised or trivialised as Miller *et al.* point out:

> between 1948 and 1996, women won 40% of Australia's gold medals at the Olympic Games despite comprising just 24% of Australia's representatives. Similarly, between 1911 and 1990 women won 35% of Australia's gold medals at the Commonwealth games in a period when they were allowed to participate in only 31% of the sports available and constituted 27% of all Australian athletes. Yet despite this astonishing performance, women's sport generally receives about 2% of Australian media sports coverage, and much of it is stereotypical, trivializing, and sexually objectifying.[70]

Perhaps a telling commentary on gender relationships within sport is the criticism of 'playing like a girl'.

Gender has been extensively studied in the context of sport and we understand how and why women are systematically marginalized and excluded.[71] This skewed playing field results in different pressures being placed on women athletes, particularly in terms of appearance and sexuality. Women, for example, are often expected to wear skimpy, tight-fitting outfits in sports where men wear baggy clothing (see both basketball and beach volleyball for example). The interaction with doping is also specific and peculiar because some performance-enhancing drugs (like testosterone and human growth hormone) can result in women becoming more like men, at least to cursory observation. This creates particular pressure on female athletes to maintain an idealized femininity (for example Florence Griffith Joyner and her spectacular fingernails). However, the female specific patterns and reasons for use of PEDs has had very little study, with the assumption being that they are the same as male use, despite the evidence we have of the very different experiences a male and a female athlete will have.

The question that sociologists ask then is this: if sport is not actually healthy or moral, why is the discourse around sport so focused upon these aspects? Sociologists answer this by arguing that sport serves other purposes in society. I have already shown how sport is about making money in a capitalist, global market. But sport and the ideas of fair play, health and morality all reinforce a particular world view.

Sport as a social value

The view of the world, how society should work, what people should do, is encapsulated by the concepts of ideology and hegemony. At their simplest these theories seek to explain how we understand our world. However, in explaining this understanding of the world, ideology and hegemony demonstrate this understanding is not neutral or natural, but shaped by social forces. Sport is thus imbued with particular values (healthy, fair and competitive) because it is important that these values continue to be propagated. Because these values are essential to the maintenance of a particular social structure – in this case capitalism – they need to be reinforced as natural and normal constantly. Sport offers a wonderful means by which to continue promulgating certain myths about society. These myths are all the more persuasive because we do not often question them or consider their validity. The attachment of these values to sport as part of a greater capitalist hegemony is also reinforced by the fact that the belief that sport embodies these ideas increases its saleability as a commodity, particularly in a period when there is an enormous focus on health and health-related issues such as childhood obesity. Because sport is seen as 'good' for the consumer, the consumer is more likely to encourage or reinforce participation, spectatorship and purchase of related goods. Thus the hegemonic understanding of sport as healthy and moral reinforces both the underlying values of capitalist society and increases the value of sport as part of consumer culture.

The fact that sport is commonly understood to be a healthy/moral activity places further emphasis on the manner in which the discourse about PEDs is constructed. If sport is understood to be healthy and moral, in common sense discourse drugs, and particularly illicitly-used drugs, are considered to be unhealthy and immoral. By overlaying these two ideas the notion of PEDs becomes a much harsher concept than it would if the common sense understanding of elite sport was closer to its reality – a highly medicalised, regime-driven activity where athletes exist in a tightly managed extreme environment.

This section has canvassed some of the key insights that sociologists offer on sports and drugs. Distilled to its essence, sociologists do not consider sport to be natural, fair or healthy. Sport is a specific activity that has arisen with the nation state and is used to further nationalist and ideological agendas. The profit motive, mediated through winning, is a central and powerful motivator in sporting competition. Sport cannot be separated from society; it is not a stand-alone institution. Finally, sport serves other purposes – that of maintaining a particular view of the world and that competition is good, inevitable and winners deserve the spoils.

What sociology needs to know

Despite the preceding discussion of sociology, which offered a complex and nuanced picture of drugs and sport, there are still further questions that need to be addressed.

I started by declaring that the sociological approach to drugs and sport consists of questioning the myths that surround sporting activity. When it comes to sport, this means considering how modern sporting competition has evolved out of play activity, and why. I then looked at how sport and capitalism have become intimately tied together, with the pursuit of victory for profit becoming a key purpose of sport. The nation state has also taken a keen role in enhancing performance to further national pride and political agendas. Two key myths were questioned, namely the ideas of fairness and health when it comes to sporting endeavours. Sport is not fair and it is not healthy – the evidence is overwhelming on these two counts.

What this questioning then led us to was an exploration of just why sport is construed the way it is today. I offered one explanation, being that sport for competition is important in maintaining capitalist, competitive ways of interacting as the only means of having a functioning society. These sociological insights point towards several focused questions that could be usefully investigated to further our understanding of sports and drugs. These questions form the basis for the research agenda outlined below.

A research agenda for sociology

Based on the argument and evidence outlined above, I have selected the following as critical to furthering our understanding of drugs *and* sport, and its cousin, drugs *in* sport:

1. amalgamating sport theory with drug theory,
2. the concept of the networked athlete,
3. prevalence rates, and
4. public perception of PED use.

In my view, knowing more about these ideas is central to informing policy responses to sport and drugs, as well as furthering our understanding of sport and the role drugs and performance-enhancing methods play.

From drugs and sport to drugs in sport

The first research priority for sociology with sport and drugs is broad and will require thoughtful, critical and carefully crafted studies. Sociologists must start to link our abundance of theory about sport and drugs together and test these theories in quantitative and qualitative studies of sport *and* drugs and drugs *in* sport. For instance, if an overriding motivation of athletes today is to win for the subsequent benefits of status and money, then sociologists need to show this. If our claims of the medicalisation of sport are to be proven, we need to get into the training rooms and observe and report upon the interactions that occur between medical staff and athletes. To support the claim that capitalism has colonised sport for the pursuit of profit, we need to demonstrate the ongoing pervasive (and possibly perverse) interaction.

The networked athlete

One avenue of research that sociologists need to pursue is the concept of the networked athlete. By that I mean that an athlete does not ever make it to elite level competition without the assistance of a host of support staff; be it coaches, doctors, nutritionists, managers, marketers, physiotherapists, acupuncturists and/or bio-mechanics to name just a few.[72] By looking at how the athlete is part of a social web we can achieve two goals. The first is a refutation of the 'lone athlete' concept in doping that seeks to test and punish just the end user. The second is that we can start to understand the micro-sociological interactions in this peculiar social world; that of the elite athlete. Waddington's argument regarding the plethora of support staff attached to athletes lends weight to this particular research agenda:

> There is now an abundance of evidence to indicate that, at least at the elite level, the drug-using athlete is normally part of a network of relationships with others, who may include team members, coaches, doctors, masseurs, trainers, managers or promoters, who are involved in supplying or administering doping substances, or in concealing their use. The highly individualistic perspective which continues to underpin the anti-doping policies adopted by organizations such as the IOC is not only based on a misunderstanding of the social relations involved in the doping process, but it also – quite wrongly – focuses exclusively on the wrongdoing of one individual while ignoring the wrongdoing of others who are heavily implicated in the use of performance-enhancing drugs.[73]

It is worth noting that Waddington was making this argument before the major Tour de France scandals and the BALCO and Madrid investigations showed that there are indeed networks of 'doping'. Further, these investigations indicate that a lone athlete model to prevention is inappropriate, inaccurate and highly unlikely to reduce doping. Social network research could also be a timely addition to the scholarship on doping issues as the National Anti-Doping Organisations (NADOs) shift function from primarily being testing, enforcement and education to investigations and rule violations. For example, ASADA points out:

> We have progressed to Anti-Doping Rule Violations which includes trafficking, investigations, failure to comply with requests for testing, positive analytical results, admission of use, not providing accurate whereabouts information, evasion, tampering. There are also much harsher rules in place for sanctioning of athlete support personnel under the rules. Athletes can now be investigated and prosecuted on information gathered.[74]

There is no doubt that testing agencies would benefit from robust social network theory research that explains how doping networks come into being, how they are maintained and by and for whom.

Prevalence

The second avenue of research that requires attention from sociologists is actual prevalence and use. We have no reliable figures on the use of PEDs, with estimates for example ranging from around 0.4% (the official FIFA incidence of positive tests in Football) to 95% (anecdotal evidence).[75] More disturbingly, these figures (both the testing agency claims and other studies) focus almost exclusively on elite athletes. What is required to further our understanding on use and prevalence is studies of elite athletes that measure use more accurately than testing. While there would be a host of ethical and methodological problems to overcome, these are not insurmountable. The second avenue of prevalence research is the use of substances at the sub-elite level. Do athletes use PEDs in under-18 (and below) competitions? What is the prevalence of use at the club level of sport amongst over-18 participants? This research would be particularly valuable as it will illuminate who is using and when – which may point to better deterrence and education methods.

Public opinion about drugs in sport

The fourth broad area of inquiry does not concern the athlete at all. While we are told by certain vested interests (testing agencies, laboratories and anti-drugs campaigners more generally) that drugs in sport are a serious problem, we do not know what the consuming public actually think of the issue. Perhaps sports consumers would not care if the Olympic 100-metre sprint was a race between the fastest men and women *and* their drug lab. The anecdotal evidence certainly points to this conclusion if we consider that fans still watch the sports most heavily mired in drug controversy (US Major League Baseball and the Tour de France for example).[76] The policy implications from such research may well be quite profound if we discover that the sport consuming public do not care or wish to know what enhancements are being used as long as they still get to enjoy the spectacle of sport.

Some final thoughts

If economics is the dismal science then sociology may be construed as the negative, critical science. It is the role of sociologists to question the way our society functions. Sport does not need more hagiography from sociology, it receives that everyday in popular discourse. Sport sociology questions what we play, how we play it and under what conditions. Critically, and perhaps the strongest contribution my discipline makes to the study of sport and drugs, is our focus on social forces and processes, not the lone drug-using athlete. All activity by the individual is construed in society, if we ignore this fact we cannot understand why an athlete will do *anything* to win.

Notes

1 Becker, 'Becoming a Marihuana User'.
2 Hargreaves, *Sporting Females: Critical Issues in the History and Sociology of Women's Sport.*
3 Dunning, 'Sociology of Sport in the Balance: Critical Reflections on Some Recent and More Enduring Trends'; Frey and Eitzen, 'Sport and Society', 504; Rowe and Lawrence, 'Framing a Critical Sports Sociology in the Age of Globalisation', 159.
4 Newman, *Sociology: Exploring the Architecture of Everyday Life*, 51.
5 C. Wright Mills, *The Sociological Imagination.*
6 Ibid., 235–6.
7 Ibid.
8 Houlihan, *Dying to Win.*
9 Armour, Jones and Kerry, 'Sport Sociology 2000', 1.
10 Marx, *The 18th Brumaire of Louis Bonaparte*, 7.
11 Armour, Jones and Kerry, 'Sport Sociology 2000', 1.
12 Frey and Eitzen, 'Sport and Society', 5.
13 Horne, *Sport in Consumer Culture*, 3; emphasis in original.
14 Miller *et al.*, *Globalization and Sport: Playing the World*, 132.
15 Horne, *Sport in Consumer Culture*, 3.
16 Frey and Eitzen, 'Sport and Society', 507.
17 Ibid., 508.
18 Ibid.
19 ABS 8686.0, Sports Industries, Australia, 2000–01.

20 ABS 4148.0, Employment in Sport and Recreation, Australia, Aug 2001.
21 Sport England, 'The Value of the Sports Economy in England', iii.
22 Horne, *Sport in Consumer Culture*, 3.
23 Ibid., drawing on Whannel, 'Book Review of Sandvoss', 481–2.
24 Horne, *Sport in Consumer Culture*; Miller *et al.*, *Globalization and Sport: Playing the World*; Hargreaves, *Sport, Power and Culture*.
25 Frey and Eitzen, 'Sport and Society', 508.
26 Waddington, 'Doping in Sport: Sociological Aspects'.
27 Horne, *Sport in Consumer Culture*, 71–94.
28 Jones and McNamee, 'Moral Reasoning, Moral Action, and the Moral Atmosphere of Sport'.
29 Ibid., 4.
30 Frey and Eitzen, 'Sport and Society', 509.
31 Horne, *Sport in Consumer Culture*.
32 Stoddart, *Saturday Afternoon Fever: Sport in Australian Culture*.
33 Ibid., 113.
34 smh.com.au, 'Chad Races in Among the Wealthy Superstars', 16 December 2004. http://www.smh.com.au/articles/2004/12/15/1102787148210.html.
35 Dart, 'Playing in a Different League'.
36 Morgan, 'Fair is Fair, Or Is It?: A Moral Consideration of the Doping Wars in American Sport'.
37 Injuryupdate.com.au, http://www.injuryupdate.com.au/forum/archive/index.php/t-568.html.
38 afl.com.au, the home page of the Australian Football League.
39 aflxmen.com. A lobby group formed to promote the plight of former AFL players, especially in regards to ongoing injury treatment.
40 Amanda Andrews, 'Branson Left Out as TV Football Rights Sell for Record'. *The Times*, May 6, 2006, http://business.timesonline.co.uk/article/0,11472-2167439,00.html.
41 Lincoln Allison, 'Faster, Stronger, Higher'. *Guardian*, August 9, 2004; Schneider, 'Cultural Nuances: Doping, Cycling and the Tour de France'.
42 Simon Longstaff, 'Hypocrisy in Gold Medal Class'. *The Australian*, January 13, 1999, http://www.ethics.org.au/things_to_read/articles_to_read/sport/article_0271.shtm.
43 Miller *et al.*, *Globalization and Sport: Playing the World*, 24.
44 Ibid., 26.
45 Hoberman, *Mortal Engines: The Science of Performance and the Dehumanisation of Sport*.
46 Hemphill, 'For the Goods of the Game: A Normative Framework for Professional Sport Management', 202.
47 Hughson, Inglis and Free, *The Uses of Sport: A Critical Study*, 125; Horne, *Sport in Consumer Culture*, 97.
48 Elias, *The Civilizing Process*, 23.
49 Hargreaves, *Sport, Power and Culture*.
50 Adair and Vamplew, *Sport in Australian History*, 93; ais.org.au, 'History of the AIS', http://www.ais.org.au/overview/history.asp; Stoddart, *Saturday Afternoon Fever: Sport in Australian Culture*, 185–92.
51 Hogan and Norton, 'The "Price" of Olympic Gold'.
52 Miller *et al.*, *Globalization and Sport: Playing the World*, 2–3.
53 Hughson, Inglis and Free, *The Uses of Sport: A Critical Study*, 124.
54 Ibid., 123–6; Stoddart, *Saturday Afternoon Fever: Sport in Australian Culture*, 158–82.
55 See Riordan, 'Sports Medicine in the Soviet Union and German Democratic Republic', for an uncritical review of East German and Soviet systems.
56 Hargreaves, *Sporting Females: Critical Issues in the History and Sociology of Women's Sport*, 225.
57 7:30 Report, 'China Moves to Clean Up its Act, but Drug-free Olympics Still in Doubt'. ABC Television, September 6, 2000, transcript available from http://www.abc.net.au/7.30/stories/s172822.htm; Mike Hurst, 'China Syndrome'. *The Daily Telegraph*, August 8, 2006; for a differing view see Hong, 'Doping and Anti-doping in Sport in China: An Analysis of Recent and Present Attitudes and Actions'.
58 UNESCO, 'Sport for Social and Human Development', http://portal.unesco.org/shs/en/ev.php-URL_ID=9534&URL_DO=DO_TOPIC&URL_SECTION=201.html.
59 Hargreaves, *Sporting Females*, 9.
60 Waddington, *Sport, Health, and Drugs: A Critical Sociological Perspective*.
61 Miller *et al.*, *Globalization and Sport: Playing the World*, 41.
62 World Anti-Doping Agency, *World Anti-Doping Code*, version 3. http://www.wada-ama.org/rtecontent/document/code_v3.pdf.
63 Houlihan, *Dying to Win*, 133–4.

64 Conrad and Potter, 'Human Growth Hormone and the Temptations of Biomedical Enhancement', 185.
65 Dingelstad *et al.*, 'The Social Construction of Drug Debates', 1832–3.
66 Waddington and Murphy, 'Drugs, Sport and Ideologies', 49–53.
67 White, 'Sick Bodies and Inequality: Class, Mortality and Morbidity', 42.
68 Cricket Australia, 'Men's Team Management', http://www.cricket.com.au/default.aspx?s = managementmens.
69 Kell, *Good Sports: Australian Sport and the Myth of the Fair Go*; or McKay, *No Pain, No Gain?*
70 Miller *et al.*, *Globalization and Sport: Playing the World*, 2.
71 Hargreaves, *Sporting Females*.
72 Waddington and Murphy, 'Drugs, Sport and Ideologies'.
73 Waddington, 'Doping in Sport: Some Issues for Medical Practitioners', 21.
74 ASADA (Australian Sport Anti-Doping Authority), personal communication, 2006.
75 Dvorak, McCrory and D'Hooghe, 'FIFA's Future Activities in the Fight Against Doping'; Morgan, 'Fair is Fair, Or Is It?: A Moral Consideration of the Doping Wars in American Sport'.
76 Allison, 'Faster, Stronger, Higher'; Schneider, 'Cultural Nuances: Doping, Cycling and the Tour de France'.

References

Adair, Daryl, and Wray Vamplew. *Sport in Australian History*. South Melbourne: Oxford University Press, 1997.

Armour, K., R. Jones, and D. Kerry. 'Sport Sociology 2000'. *Sociology of Sport Online*, 2000. http://physed.otago.ac.nz/sosol/home.html.

Becker, Howard S. 'Becoming a Marihuana User'. *The American Journal of Sociology* 59, no. 3 (1953): 235–42.

Conrad, Peter, and Deborah Potter. 'Human Growth Hormone and the Temptations of Biomedical Enhancement'. *Sociology of Health Illness* 26, no. 2 (2004): 184–215.

Dart, Tony. 'Playing in a Different League'. In *Football in the Digital Age: Whose Game is it Anyway?* edited by Sean Hamil, Jonathan Michie, Christine Oughton, and Steven Warby, 144–50. Edinburgh: Mainstream, 2000.

Dingelstad, David, Richard Gosden, Brian Martin, and Nickolas Vakas. 'The Social Construction of Drug Debates'. *Social Science and Medicine* 43, no. 12 (1996): 1829–38.

Dunning, Eric. 'Sociology of Sport in the Balance: Critical Reflections on Some Recent and More Enduring Trends'. Paper presented at the 28th Annual Conference of the Social History Society, Leicester, 2003.

Dvorak, J., P. McCrory, and M. D'Hooghe. 'FIFA's Future Activities in the Fight Against Doping'. *British Journal of Sports Medicine* 40, Supp. 1 (2006): 158–59.

Elias, Norbert. *The Civilizing Process*. Oxford: Blackwell, 1986.

Frey, James H., and Stanley D. Eitzen. 'Sport and Society'. *Annual Review of Sociology* 17 (1991): 503–22.

Hargreaves, Jennifer. *Sporting Females: Critical Issues in the History and Sociology of Women's Sport*. London: Routledge, 1994.

Hargreaves, John. *Sport, Power and Culture*. Cambridge: Polity Press, 1986.

Hemphill, Dennis. (1997) 'For the Goods of the Game: A Normative Framework for Professional Sport Management'. In *Advances in the Management of Australian and New Zealand Sport*, 192–207. Proceedings of the 2nd Annual Sport Management Association of Australia and New Zealand Conference, 192–207. Burwood: Sport Management Association of Australia and New Zealand, 1996.

Hoberman, John. *Mortal Engines: The Science of Performance and the Dehumanisation of Sport*. New York: The Blackburn Press, 1992.

Hogan, K., and K. Norton. 'The "Price" of Olympic Gold'. *Journal of Science and Medicine in Sport* 3, no. 2 (June 2000): 203–18.

Hong, Fan. 'Doping and Anti-doping in Sport in China: An Analysis of Recent and Present Attitudes and Actions'. *Sport in Society* 9, no. 2 (2006): 314–33.

Horne, John. *Sport in Consumer Culture*. Houndmills: Palgrave, 2006.

Houlihan, Barrie. *Dying to Win*, 2nd ed. Strasbourg: Council of Europe Publishing, 2002.

Hughson, J., D. Inglis, and M. Free. *The Uses of Sport: A Critical Study*. New York: Routledge, 2005.

Jones, C., and Mike McNamee. 'Moral Reasoning, Moral Action, and the Moral Atmosphere of Sport'. *Sport, Education and Society* 5, no. 2 (2000): 131–47.

Kell, Peter. *Good Sports: Australian Sport and the Myth of the Fair Go*. Annandale: Pluto, 2000.

Marx, Karl. *The 18th Brumaire of Louis Bonaparte*. London: The Electric Book Company, 2001 [1852].

McKay, Jim. *No Pain, No Gain?* Sydney: Prentice Hall, 1991.

Miller, T., G. Lawrence, J. McKay, and D. Rowe. *Globalization and Sport: Playing the World*. London: Sage, 2001.

Mills, C. Wright. *The Sociological Imagination*. Harmondsworth: Penguin, 1973.

Morgan, William J. 'Fair is Fair, Or Is It?: A Moral Consideration of the Doping Wars in American Sport'. *Sport and Society* 9, no. 2 (2006): 177–98.

Newman, David M. *Sociology: Exploring the Architecture of Everyday Life*, 3rd ed. Thousand Oaks, CA: Pine Forge Press, 1995.

Riordan, Jim. 'Sports Medicine in the Soviet Union and German Democratic Republic'. *Social Science and Medicine* 25, no. 1 (1987): 19–26.

Rowe, David, and Geoffrey Lawrence. 'Framing a Critical Sports Sociology in the Age of Globalisation'. In *Tourism, Leisure, Sport: Critical Perspectives*, edited by David Rowe and Geoffrey Lawrence, 159–69. Rydalmere, NSW: Hodder, 1998.

Schneider, Angela J. 'Cultural Nuances: Doping, Cycling and the Tour de France'. *Sport in Society* 9, no. 2 (2006): 212–26.

Sport England. 'The Value of the Sports Economy in England'. Final Report, June 2003. Cambridge: Cambridge Econometrics.

Stoddart, Brian. *Saturday Afternoon Fever: Sport in Australian Culture*. North Ryde, NSW: Angus and Robertson, 1986.

Waddington, Ivan. 'Doping in Sport: Sociological Aspects'. Paper presented to a special meeting of the European Commission called to investigate doping in sport, Brussels, 1999. http://www.chester.ac.uk/ccrss/research.html#ivan.

Waddington, Ivan. *Sport, Health, and Drugs: A Critical Sociological Perspective*. London: E & FN Spon, 2000.

Waddington, Ivan. 'Doping in Sport: Some Issues for Medical Practitioners'. Lecture at the Leiden International Medical Students Congress, University of Leiden Medical School, Netherlands, March, 2001. www.ucd.ie/css/papers/leiden%20paper.pdf.

Waddington, Ivan, and Patrick Murphy. 'Drugs, Sport and Ideologies'. In *Sport and Leisure in the Civilizing Process*, edited by Eric Dunning and Chris Rojek, 36–64. London: MacMillan, 1992.

Whannel, G. 'Book Review of Sandvoss'. *British Journal of Sociology* 55, no. 3 (2004): 481–2.

White, Kevin. 'Sick Bodies and Inequality: Class, Mortality and Morbidity'. In *Inequality in Australia*, edited by A. Greig, F. Lewins and K. White, 39–56. Melbourne: Cambridge, 2003.

The economics of drugs in sport

Keiran Sharpe

School of Business, UNSW@ADFA, Canberra, Australia

This essay explains the approach that economists take when explaining the phenomenon of drug-taking in sport. The economic method models such drug-taking as a rational activity in which athletes respond to the existing incentives. The 'solution' to the drugs in sport problem is to alter the incentives under which athletes operate. The essay notes that there are two means for implementing such alterations. The first is via regulation, and the second is via the operation of market forces within the market for different sports. The latter modality is naturally suggested as the preferred one by the economic method. However, as the essay reports, the full analysis of this issue has not been completed, so the essay is agnostic on the matter of the optimal manner for changing the incentives under which athletes operate.

In the economic analysis of drugs in sport, drug taking is explained as a rational activity, and the effectiveness of alternative drug abatement regimes is explained in terms of the incentives they provide for rational players not to take drugs. While existing models in the economics literature adequately explicate the arguments for the taking of drugs by contestants in sports, there are few models that expand upon the comparative merits of alternative schemata for abating drug use. This is to say that the incentive effects of alternative regimes are not well attested, and, *a fortiori*, the social welfare implications of the different abatement regimes are relatively unknown. Certainly, there is no general theory of drug use and abatement in sports. This essay suggests a possible way forward for economic research on this subject.

How economics sees the world

As a prelude to the discussion that follows, it's worth noting that economics uses mathematical notation and some specific jargon to describe the world. These are unavoidable and are deployed below; however, prose accounts are also given for the mathematically disinterested reader.

Economics is the study of rational behaviour; which is to say it's the study of the way in which reasoning persons settle upon actions in pursuit of the aims they have. As such, it is a teleological method and therefore distinct from the other social sciences, in which it's generally assumed that people are in the grip of external forces that they cannot wilfully apprehend (such as psychological, social and cultural forces).

Specifically, economics supposes that each person – or 'agent' in the argot – has a well-defined utility function, $U(\mathbf{x})$, which specifies the agent's preferences over the various outcomes he values. This is to say that the $U(\mathbf{x})$ function indicates how much utility the agent gets from each amount of the goods given in the vector (or 'list'), $\mathbf{x}$. The agent also faces a set of constraints (c), and $g(\mathbf{x}) \leq c$, which determines the range of options he has. (The $\mathbf{x}$ in $U(\mathbf{x})$ and $g(\mathbf{x})$ indicates the set of goods the person can aim at attaining.) The agent then attempts to solve the following problem. Choose $\mathbf{x}$ so as to:

$$\text{maximize } U(\mathbf{x})$$

$$\text{subject to}: \ g(\mathbf{x}) \leq c$$

In the context of sports competition, the agent might want to maximize his rank, but he is constrained in this pursuit by his naturally given talents, the availability of time, a limited training budget and, of course, the behaviour of his competitors. Given those constraints, the athlete works out a strategy that maximizes his chances of winning (or at least of doing the best he can).

There are at least two possible uses of economic models of the type just described. The first is to take them as descriptive of the way actual persons behave; the other is to take them as determining the norms of rational conduct.

With regard to the first usage, there is plenty of criticism that economics is 'unrealistic' in the assumptions it makes and, therefore, in the conclusions that it reaches. There is an old folk wisdom that this is generally the case; and there is also, by now, an extensive experimental literature which shows that people do not generally behave in a rational way. The literature on this matter was initiated by the work of Kahneman and Tversky amongst others, and is now very diverse.[1]

Following the largely negative findings of the empirical research, there has been a tendency to think of economics theory as rather determining what it means for a person to be rational; that is, as determining the norms of rational conduct. The argument here is that although economics has difficulty explaining what people actually do, it can explain what they would do were they rational – that is to say, it can propose some kind of rational ideal to set against the reality of people's bumbling along.

This bifurcation into descriptive – or 'positive' theory – and normative theory, however, is largely based on an epistemological error. All theory necessarily involves some degree of idealization or abstraction, and all theories adopt some kind of idealized/abstracted entities which are reified in the theories' models (one thinks here, for example, of the role that the centre of mass plays in Newtonian mechanics). The question, then, is not whether the world strictly conforms to the picture generated by the models, but whether the models predict (or retrodict) changes in the world to a sufficient order of approximation given an initial state of play. Adapting this thought to the current context means that economics does not require people to be rational all of the time, or even most of the time; it only requires that people be mostly rational most of the time; and that is probably a workable hypothesis. In any event, it's the model of agency we shall be using here to investigate some of the issues surrounding the use of drugs in sport.

What economics has done

Theoretical context

There are two things to note about the economics of drugs in sport. The first is that it naturally fits into the sub-discipline of the theory of information and incentives, which overlaps with the theory of games; and the second is that there is very little direct research on the topic of why athletes take performance-enhancing drugs.[2] Given the natural fit of the phenomenon with existing analytical methods it is a little surprising that so little research has been done in the area, and it suggests that there is some room for future research on this topic.

The theory of incentives concerns, as the name suggests, the topic of how economic agents can be provided with the right incentives to act in various ways. There are many and various applications of the theory, but a large area of analysis involves the investigation of the so-called 'principal-agent problem'. This arises when one player, the principal, would like the other, the agent, to act in a particular way, but, in the most interesting cases, cannot directly observe the way in which the agent behaves. This is to say that there is an asymmetry of information between the two players. Hence, the principal must construct some mechanism that will induce or 'incentivize' the agent to act in the desired manner. Examples occur in the insurance industry where the principal – the insurer – cannot observe the insuree's behaviour, but can provide mechanisms to abate moral hazard (by such things as no-claims bonuses, excesses, exclusions and the like); or in employment, where the owner – the principal – cannot observe the workforce's effort, but knows that successful performance is correlated with effort, and so offers performance bonuses; and so on.

One kind of incentive mechanism is the 'promotion tournament' whereby effort is induced by the selection of only the top-ranked competitors for promotion. The incentive effects of such tournaments mimic those of ordinary sports competitions.[3] Happily, the economics of the way in which such tournaments work is relatively well understood; and, since the operation of the economic models that describe such tournaments is directly germane to our discussion, it is worthwhile considering a simple example.

A model: a verbal account

We here present a model of how economists think competitors behave, and what motivates them to cheat. In the next section, we present a more formal version of the argument given in this section. The next section can accordingly be passed over by the mathematically disinterested reader.

In any given contest, we suppose that there are N players, each of whom wants to increase the odds of their winning, and who also benefit from the 'regard' or esteem in which the sport is held. The odds of winning and the state of regard of the sport depend on the decisions and conduct of any given player himself and of all the other players of the sport. The more other players decide not to cheat, the higher is the regard in which the sport is held by the public. Consequently, the greater are the chances of winning for a given player. Hence, the decisions of other players not to cheat are both directly and indirectly beneficial to the player. However, in determining how he should behave, a competitor faces a dilemma, for a decision not to cheat increases the regard of the sport relative to the situation that would arise were they to decide to cheat, but it reduces the relative odds of winning. This is the nub of the problem confronting the athlete – and the sports regulator trying to reduce the incidence of cheating in the sport.

This characterization of the situation confronting the players suggests that they are engaged in a de facto 'referendum' on the sport when they decide whether or not to cheat. Specifically, the referendum asks: would you prefer to participate in a clean sport and pay the price of doing so by not taking drugs yourself? The player 'votes' when they decide whether to cheat or not.

It turns out that if three conditions are met, sufficient numbers of players elect to cheat, so making the sport 'drug-tainted'. The three conditions are: 1) strategic complementarity, 2) sure weak link, and, 3) epidemic weakness. *Strategic complementarity* arises just in the case when a critical number of decisions to cheat by others means that the payoff to any one player in deciding not to cheat is less than the payoff to cheating. In other words, there is some level of cheating – or perceived cheating – by others that induces each athlete to cheat. Every player has their price, so to speak, and there are no Kantians amongst sportsmen. The *sure weak link* condition is met if there is a critical subset of players who decide to cheat regardless of how many others decide to cheat. This is to say that someone always cheats. *Epidemic weakness* states that if a certain subset of players is thought to cheat, then another subset also decide to cheat, and if these two subsets are thought to cheat, then so will a further subset of players, and so on.

If these three conditions are satisfied, we can then demonstrate that an 'epidemic' of cheating will occur. Moreover, if cheating is widespread, it must be the case that some such epidemic has occurred. This epidemic, of course, is not driven by biological or any other deterministic forces; rather, it is driven by the rationality of the players themselves. It occurs because some players cheat regardless of the conduct of others and because others start to cheat in response, and yet more others cheat in response to this 'second round' of cheating and so on, until cheating is endemic. In other words, the epidemic occurs because each rational player responds rationally to the conduct of others, who are themselves behaving rationally. It is just this kind of epidemic which National Anti-Doping Organisations (NADOs) are trying to manage in their 'war against drugs in sport'. The institutional structures that regulatory agencies might set up in order to wage this war are discussed below (and, as remarked earlier, the mathematically disinclined reader ought to proceed directly to that section).

A model: a mathematical account

We begin by supposing that there are $i = 1, \ldots, N$ players in a contest and that each player gets utility from just two goods: the probability of winning, p^i, and the regard with which the sport is held, R^i. For all players, utility increases with increases in the regard in which the sport is held and in the probability of winning. That is, in the terms of the calculus, we have: $u^i = u^i(R^i, p^i)$, with: $\partial u^i/\partial R^i > 0$ and $\partial u^i/\partial p^i > 0 \; \forall i$.

Both the regard of the sport and the probability of winning are functions of the decision of the agent, and the decisions of all the other agents, to cheat or not. That is, $R^i = R^i(\mathrm{e}^i, \mathbf{e}^{-i})$ and $p^i = p^i(\mathrm{e}^i, \mathbf{e}^{-i})$, where $e^i \in \{0, 1\} = \{$'cheat', 'don't cheat'$\} =$ the options of cheating or not cheating for player *i*, and $\mathbf{e}^{-i}$ is the $N - 1$ vector of such decisions by the other agents. If it doesn't matter to player *i* what any other individual decides to do, but only how many other players choose to cheat or not, then the two functions simplify to: $R^i = R^i(\mathrm{e}^i, \mathbf{E}^{-i})$ and $p^i = p^i(\mathrm{e}^i, \mathbf{E}^{-i})$ where $\mathbf{E}^{-i} = \sum_{-i} \mathrm{e}^{-i} =$ the summation of the decisions of all athletes except competitor *i* (obviously this is a scalar). It's then reasonable to suppose that: $\Delta R^i/\Delta \mathbf{E}^{-i} > 0$ and $\Delta p^i/\Delta \mathbf{E}^{-i} > 0$; i.e. the more the other competitors decide not to cheat, the higher is the regard in which the sport is held and the greater are the chances of winning. Hence, the decisions of other players not to cheat indirectly increases the utility of any given competitor by increasing the utility obtained from both R^i and p^i. However, in determining how he should behave, competitor *i* faces a dilemma, for a decision not to cheat increases the regard of the sport relative to the situation that would arise were they to decide to cheat, but it reduces the relative odds of winning. Formally, the situation is: $R^i(1|\mathbf{E}^{-i}) > R^i(0|\mathbf{E}^{-i})$ and $p^i(1|\mathbf{E}^{-i}) < p^i(0|\mathbf{E}^{-i})$. This characterizes the essential conundrum confronting the athlete.

This representation of the decision problem confronting the athlete is tantamount to suggesting that the players are involved in a kind of 'referendum' on the sport they play. Formally, the referendum is a mapping, $\mathrm{M} : \{0, 1\}_{i=1}^{i=N} \rightarrow \mathbf{R}^{2N}$, which takes the expressed 'votes' (i.e. the decisions to cheat or not) of the athletes to the quantity of regard and the probability of winning of each of the *N* competitors. The existence of the vector-valued function, $\mathrm{M}(\mathbf{e})$, mapping the athletes' 'votes' to the level of regard and the odds of winning, implies that each athlete has an indirect utility function, $\mathrm{v}^i(\mathrm{e}^i, \mathbf{e}^{-i}) = \mathrm{u}^i(\mathrm{M}(\mathrm{e}^i, \mathbf{e}^{-i}))$ (i.e. the value of a vote, e^i, to athlete *i* depends on e^i itself and on the votes of all the other sportsmen given by the $N - 1$ vector, $\mathbf{e}^{-i}$). Each athlete *i* then has the problem: max $\mathrm{v}^i(\mathrm{e}^i, \mathbf{e}^{-i})$. An equilibrium of the 'to-cheat-or-not-to-cheat' referendum is a state (S) where all the players simultaneously attain a maximum; i.e.: $S = \{\mathbf{e} \in \{0, 1\}_{i=1}^{i=N} | \max v^i(e^i, e^{-i}) \forall i\}$.

This construction of the problem facing athletes leads us to ask how it is that they vote, and, in particular, under what conditions they elect to cheat. The following three conditions and the subsequent propositions give us some guidance on this matter.

Let the voting mechanism, $M(\cdot)$, satisfy:

(1) *strategic complementarity:* $\exists \hat{E}^{-i} : v^i(1|\mathbf{E}^{-i} \leq \hat{E}^{-i}) < v^i(0|\mathbf{E}^{-i} \leq \hat{E}^{-i}) \; \forall i$
(which has the interpretation: there exists a critical number of 0 votes by others such that the payoff to *i*'s deciding not to cheat is less than the payoff to cheating);

(2) *sure weak link:* $E[v^N(1)] < E[v^N(0)]$
(which has the interpretation: for athlete *N*, the expected value of switching from the decision not to cheat to cheating, given only knowledge of $M(\cdot)$, is greater than zero (where we note that $E[\cdot]$ is the expectation operator));

(3) *epidemic weakness:* $\exists \{E[v^i(\cdot)]\}_{i=1}^{i=N-1} : E[v^{i+1}(1)] < E[v^{i+1}(0) => E[v^i(1)] < E[v^i(0)]$
(which has the interpretation: there exists a sequence $1, \ldots, i, \ldots, N-1$ such that if it pays athlete $i+1$ to cheat, then it pays athlete i to cheat also).

Strategic complementarity says that each athlete has an incentive to cheat if sufficient others do so. The reason for this is that, once that threshold is reached, the loss of utility caused by the damage he does to the sport is outweighed by the increase in utility he obtains by cheating. *Sure weak link* says that someone will certainly cheat either because he does not have much regard for the sport (or does not care about the regard others have for the sport) or because, while he does have regard for the sport, he thinks someone else will cheat, and so is incentivized to cheat himself. *Epidemic weakness* says that if athlete *i* thinks that athlete $i+1$ will cheat, then it pays *i* to cheat as well (since his critical threshold will then be attained). These assumptions are sufficiently general to characterize Prisoner's Dilemma and Common Assurance games, and games with iterated dominant solutions; in short, these assumptions characterize the class of games known as 'social dilemmas'. With that in mind, we can then state the following results.

Proposition 1. If (1) – (3) hold then all athletes vote 0 (i.e. all athletes cheat).

Proof. We begin by observing that (2) & (3) $\Rightarrow$ (1) since if $\neg$ (1) it is not possible that $E[v^i(1)] < E[v^i(0)] \; \forall i$. Now take agent N. $e^N = 0$ by (2). But then $e^{N-1} = 0$; $e^{N-2} = 0$; and so on, by (3). Therefore, $e^i = 0 \; \forall i$. □

Corollary. (1) $v^i(0|\mathbf{E}^{-i} = 0) > v^i(1|\mathbf{E}^{-i} = 0) \forall i => \{0\}_{i=1}^{i=N} \in S$.

It's worth remarking that assumption (2) – the existence of a sure weak link – may hold either because of straightforward dominance in payoffs for athlete *N* (i.e. $\hat{\mathbf{E}}^{-N} = 0$); or because of risk dominance considerations (i.e., although $\hat{\mathbf{E}}^{-N} > 0$, athlete *N* votes $e^N = 0$ (i.e. votes to cheat) out of fear that sufficient others will set $e^i = 0$). If the former situation holds true, then it is the case that some athletes simply do not care for the regard in which the sport is held, and will cheat regardless, so setting off the chain reaction of cheating in the sport. The possibility of the latter case is important as it gives some cause for optimism that means might be found to choke off the chain reaction; the reason for this is that, in this latter case, all the athletes are 'honourable' in the sense that they would prefer not to cheat – and would not cheat in a world of perfect information. They only end up doing so out of fear that others will. In this latter case – that is, if (2) does hold because of 'risk dominance' considerations – then we have two equilibria: $\{1\}_{i=1}^{i=N}, \{0\}_{i=1}^{i=N} \in S$, where $\{1\}_{i=1}^{i=N}$ Pareto dominates $\{0\}_{i=1}^{i=N}$. This is to say that a no-one-cheats equilibrium exists and is preferred by all players to the 'everyone-cheats' equilibrium. However, the former outcome is unstable and the latter is stable owing to (2) (the existence of a weak link) and (3) (epidemic weakness). Hence, the 'collective' decision to cheat is made even though it is Pareto dominated (i.e. is dispreferred to no cheating by everyone).

We also have the following proposition.

Proposition 2. If $e^i = 0\ \forall i\ \&\ E[v^i(1|e^N = 1)] > E[v^i(0|e^N = 1)]$ for $i = 1, \ldots, N-1$, then (1)–(3) hold.

Proof. If $\neg$ (2), $S = \{1\}_N$; if $\neg$ (1), $e^i = 1$ dominates for some i; if $\neg$ (3); $e^i = 1$ dominates for some i. So (1) – (3) hold. □

The effect of propositions 1 and 2 is the following: widespread cheating can be understood as a kind of rational epidemic caused by the strategic complementarity of athletes' actions which creates an incentive to cheat if sufficient others are thought to do so. The logic of this kind of model is well understood and widely attested in the economic literature.[4] And it raises the question: how can we stop the epidemic of cheating given the inherent incentive to cheat in tournaments? Unfortunately, the theoretical and empirical economics of the answer to this question are less well understood.

What economics needs to know

There are two basic mechanisms for attempting to abate the tendency to cheat by taking drugs: the first is external regulation, i.e. regulation by investigative bodies that are external to the corps of athletes themselves and which are therefore not subject to the 'perverse' incentives to cheat described in the above model; the second involves some degree of self-regulation by the corps of athletes, where the athletes are presumed to be responsive to the concerns of spectators and others who help determine the degree of regard in which the sport is held.[5]

Regulation external to sport

Regulation works to reduce the incentive to cheat by reducing the probability of succeeding by cheating, and does so by increasing the probability of being caught if one cheats and by reducing the payoff if one wins by cheating (and is caught); that is, incentive-based deterrence. (This is to say, it attempts to alter the $p^i(e^i, \mathbf{E}^{-i})$ function by reducing $\Delta p^i/\Delta e^i$.) If all else were equal, this would certainly work to cause some abatement of the endemic tendency to cheat; however, the introduction of regulation tends to bring problematic baggage of its own.

The first difficulty with regulation is that it tends to be expensive, bureaucratic and legalistic. The direct expense of regulation is a matter of public record since the bodies are public agencies; however, less well known are the opportunity costs. This is to say that the relative costs and benefits of alternative schemata of drug-use abatement have not been systematically assessed, so that the relative cost-effectiveness of regulation is not known. Hence, we don't currently know whether regulation is the most effective method for reducing any given level of drug use or whether some other, as yet untried, *modus operandi* is better. Nor do we know the level of drug use that is tolerable to society; which is to say that we do not currently know how much society is willing to expend on drug-abatement in sports relative to, say, the building of schools or of hospitals or the taking of tax cuts. In the jargon of the given discipline, the welfare economics of drug abatement has thus far been inadequately analysed. Because we do not know which method is the most cost effective means of abating drug use in sports, and because we do not even know how much society is willing to spend on the abatement of drug use relative to other kinds of expenditure, we cannot know the opportunity costs of the current regulatory regimes. This is a major lacuna that needs to be filled.

The bureaucratic nature of external regulation is known to economists to bring its own problems, of which, two are well known. The first is the tendency of bureaucracies to become overly large as managers inflate the nature of the problem they have to deal with in order to increase their call on fiscal resources. This is done in order to increase the power and prestige that come from managing a larger civil service organization.[6] In the current context this means that there is a natural tendency to perceive any given level of drug use as excessive, where 'excessive' here means in excess of the marginal net social benefits of eliminating it; and this perception overstates the real social costs of marginal drug use. One sees examples of this mentality in the draconian regulation of commonly used and historically licit drugs such as tobacco today or alcohol during the period of the validity of the Eighteenth Amendment in the United States; and there is no reason to think that, once created, sports governing bodies (SGBs) and NADOs (including WADA) will be any less inclined to push for measures that increase their call on budgetary resources in excess of the social benefits that might be brought about by the use of those resources to abate drug usage at the margin. In fact, theory suggests just the reverse; that is to say, they would seek to increase their resource allocation and power irrespective of programme or policy success.

There is another problem with the incentive structures inherent in bureaucracies: bureaucracies generally have less incentive to catch malfeasance than miscreants have to avoid being caught. This may not be a problem when the resources of the state and the economies of scale of law enforcement are sufficiently large relative to those available to the miscreants to create a counter-asymmetry to the incentive effect; but it is more problematic when the allocation of resources is not so much in favour of the state, as is the case of drug use in sport. Again, the question is begged about the relative costs and benefits of the bureaucratic/regulatory approach vis-à-vis other methods of enforcement.

The second species of difficulty with regulation lies in the particular way in which external regulation typically works. Generally speaking, regulation works by listing banned substances and testing competitors on a random basis for those substances – a methodology known as the negative list system (promulgated by the WADC). The difficulty with such an approach is that it simply shifts the locus of cheating from the covert use of known performance-enhancing substances to the use of substances yet to be proscribed. Hence, the negative list system supplants one incentive-to-cheat mechanism with another. Of course, this would not be a problem if the ability to act on the new incentives were low, but the evidence seems to be that it is not – which is to say that the existence of an extensive and profitable substance-inventing industry is evidence (e.g. BALCO), *ipso facto*, that it pays to subvert the regulatory system. In fact, by shifting the incentive to cheat 'upstream', the negative list system creates a further distortion in the competition amongst athletes since only wealthier athletes are able to afford 'exotic' doping regimens.[7] Hence, the distribution of gains from participating in sports is shifted towards athletes from the wealthier nations.

All this suggests that an alternative approach to government regulation might be preferred. What follows is speculative, but it is implicitly suggested by the economic approach.

Alternative external regulation

If we return to the specification of the utility function of the typical athlete, we recall that: $u^i = u^i(R^i, p^i)$, i.e. utility is a function both of the regard in which the sport is held and of the odds of winning. The former variable we have left rather vague – it could represent the subjective sense of sportsmanship and integrity of the athlete themself, or it could represent the regard in which others hold the sport. In this latter case, one supposes that more mercenary motives might be in play for the athlete. For example, he might think that the greater is the regard in which the sport is held as a 'clean' (i.e. drug-free) sport by the paying public (the view currently assumed to prevail, although the author was unable to uncover evidence that this is the case), the more likely it is that they'll be interested in spectating the sport; consequently, the greater will be the overall takings of the sport, and the greater their own earnings will be. If that is indeed the case, it may be more effective to abate drug use in sport by working through the impact on reputation (i.e. the $R^i(\mathrm{e}^i, \mathbf{E}^{-i})$ function) rather than upon the likelihood of getting caught (i.e. the $p^i(\mathrm{e}^i, \mathbf{E}^{-i})$ function). As we've seen, it is via this latter avenue that the regulatory approach works.

An alternative approach might then work as follows. The government might kick things off, so to speak, by educating the public – especially those members of it who are actively engaged in sporting activities – on the relative virtues of 'clean' sports conduct (which appears to be current practice). This has an immediate effect of increasing the marginal desire of players to participate in, and to observe, clean sports (i.e. this will increase $\Delta R^i/\Delta \mathbf{e}^i$) and, thereby, will directly abate some drug use. Such a programme will have a proportionately greater impact the more importantly the athlete's value 'regard' or esteem over winning. Hence, the greatest impact will be on amateur sporting activity. If the aim of the government is to maximize overall societal health by minimizing deleterious drug use, this programme may be sufficient. However, it is unlikely to be sufficient to abate drug use in highly professional sports since the emphasis that athletes place on winning is so much the greater because the relative gains from doing so are so high. So, supplementary programmes will have to come in to play at that level. However, this approach may have some influence at the non-elite level.

Regulation internal to sports

The second part of an alternative approach that is suggested by the economics literature is to incentivize professional sportsmen to report on each other. A necessary, but likely insufficient, condition for such reporting is that the public support the goal of reducing drug use. This is necessary as, otherwise, there would be no source of gain for the sport as a whole from drug abatement, nor, *a fortiori*, for the individual (reporting) sportsman. In other words, if the public refuses to pay to watch clean rather than dirty sports then there is no market demand to pay for drug abatement. However, even if such demand for relatively clean sports does exist, it's unlikely to be sufficient to incentivize effective peer reporting of drug cheats for the following reason. The gains of increased regard that are brought about by peer reporting accrue to the sport as a whole and are only disbursed to the player himself in an indirect and marginal manner. The gains from successful cheating, however, are direct and of the first order. This is to say that the costs of investigating the conduct of suspected cheats are high for an individual sportsman to bear, yet the gains from successful exposure accrue to all the other clean players in the sport, and this weakens the incentive for any individual athlete to investigate and expose the cheating of others ('why should I solely bear the costs of investigation and prosecution of drug cheats when the benefits accrue to everyone in the sport?'). On the other hand, players who are cheating have a much stronger incentive to avoid being caught since they fully bear the costs of being exposed. Players therefore have a greater incentive to cover up their own illicit drug use than they have to obtain sufficient evidence on their co-sportsmen to 'blow the whistle' with credibility. Consequently, a 'gap' arises between what is good for a sport as a whole and what is good for the individual sportsperson; correspondingly, the incentive to report is weak.

In the jargon of economics, we say that there are unexploited positive externalities in this case. This is to say that there exist unexploited opportunities for players to generate benefits for all the athletes within a given sport by reporting on cheats. The problem then becomes one of building appropriate institutions that spread the costs of investigating cheating in a given sport, or a set of sporting activities, over all the participants in the sport(s), thereby lowering the costs of whistle blowing for any one athlete. Such an institutional structure mimics the way in which the criminal law is enforced. In this latter case, the costs to any one citizen – or even any small subset of citizens – of enforcing the law on their own are too high, so society taxes all citizens to establish a police force and a judicial system in order to spread the costs of investigating and prosecuting criminals. The only requirement of citizens is that they be truthful witnesses to crimes and that they report the crimes they see. Under such an arrangement, the benefits of the rule of law accrue to each law-abiding citizen, while the costs are spread over all such citizens. This institutional structure is economically efficient since it generates a net social benefit at low individual cost; and, as we say in economics, it does so by 'internalizing the externality' that arises from living under the rule of law. Equally, we say it stops 'free riding' by spreading the costs of maintaining the rule of law across all the society's members.

Creating a system of regulation internal to sports

The question then arises as to what such an institutional structure looks like in the context of the regulation of drugs in sport. Fortunately, we know what such a structure looks like as it already exists in multifarious forms. Sports naturally attempt to secure the gains of 'law enforcement' by establishing peak bodies that determine relevant codes of ethics, fix the punishments for the breaches of those codes, and investigate reported abusive behaviour within the various sports (e.g. NADOs, WADA, SGBs, NFs, IFs, *etc*). Each peak body has an incentive to encourage players to report drug usage since doing so increases the regard in which the sport is held (subject to a caveat which is discussed below), and, thereby, increases the sport's aggregate purse (assuming that spectators prefer to watch 'drug-free' rather than 'drug-affected' contests). Players themselves then have an incentive to report usage too since the costs of investigating and sustaining credible complaints against co-sportspeople are spread over the whole corps of athletes in the sport. Reporting players will also obtain a 'windfall' gain from the elimination of players credibly 'convicted' of drug usage since their chances of winning contests will have improved.[8] Of course, this system of reporting creates an incentive to accuse co-sportsmen falsely in order to secure the windfall gain. To counter this consequence of relying on peer reportage, the making of complaints that are not based on adequate *prima facie* evidence may be punished on the grounds of their being vexatious, as is standard practice in legal codes.

The advantages of such a system of invigilation are threefold. First, by operating through the influence of the regard or esteem in which the sport is held by the (paying) public, the incentives to report drug usage are more closely aligned with the interests of the spectating public than is the case for bureaucracies. This is so because it only pays a peak body to proscribe and investigate drug usage that the public is concerned about, rather than the ingestion of every single performance-enhancing chemical compound (and, as we've mentioned earlier, the sports regulation bureaucracy has an inherent incentive to extend proscription beyond the scope of public interest – see the reference to the Niskanen paper). To that extent, society's attitudes to the costs and benefits of drug usage might be better reflected in the ethical codes of practice that are enforced by peak bodies than they are in the regulations of external government agencies.

Second, since players might generally be expected to be better informed about doping practices than external agencies, the discovery of such behaviour ought generally to be better once players are incentivized to report such usage. Players will be incentivized to abate drug usage in ways that bureaucrats are not if they are cognizant of the net benefits to the sport (and therefore to themselves) of their doing so. This is to say that athletes will be motivated to report drug cheats if they can see that public support and monetary demand for the sport is increased if the sport is clean. Civil servants, on the other hand, are not so directly incentivized to expose drug cheats. Finally, since enforcement is, in the first instance, undertaken by (profit maximizing) peak bodies, the system is less costly to the state, and might generally be expected to be less costly overall than the alternative bureaucratic/regulatory regime. This is because peak bodies have a greater incentive to keep costs down (because they have less call on fiscal resources than does the state, and because cost increases directly eat into the net income of the participants of the sport).

The major difficulty with the mooted alternative is that it creates another incentive problem. For sports codes compete against each other, so that if the public is generally opposed to drug usage, there's an incentive of the peak bodies to hide such drug usage as is found so as not to harm the sport's reputation vis-à-vis other codes. In economics, this kind of 'knock-on' effect is well understood, and is a consequence of agents living in a 'second-best' world – i.e. in a world in which the constraints on reaching a first-best world are insurmountable. The world in which athletes compete is second best in this sense because there is always an incentive to cheat one way or another since the gains from doing so successfully are so great, and information about who is cheating is never perfect.

There are at least two possible solutions to this 'second best' problem. The first is for the government to audit the different sports bodies. Such audits would involve public assessments of the sports' ethical codes and the resources dedicated to the enforcement of those codes, and might be accompanied by occasional investigations by the governmental enforcement agency into particular instances of breaches of those codes. This approach is effectively a public information exercise combined with a naming and shaming regime which is triggered in those cases where shortfalls in peak body performance are uncovered. Again, although there is no formal modelling of the effectiveness of such an approach, economic theory suggests that it might be cost-effective.

An alternative, and potentially cheaper, solution to the second best problem created by the competition between peak bodies is to rely on the Fourth Estate to undertake the auditing of those bodies' performances. Again, if the public is genuinely concerned about drug usage, it is in the interests of the media to thoroughly investigate apparent breaches of the codes of ethics under which the peak bodies purport to operate. Fear of adverse reporting by the media and the consequent knock-on effects on spectator interest may be the most cost-effective deterrent to the development of a permissive drug culture in sport.

A final word on alternative regulation

All this is of course, highly speculative, and we might conclude this section by reinforcing the reader's scepticism of both methods for abating drug use in sport – neither the existing regulatory system nor the alternative sketched above is convincingly superior to the other, nor is either evidently superior to any further regime that might be proposed. This is just the point with which we want to leave this section: the economics of the relative costs and benefits of alternative drug abatement regimes is under-attested, and constitutes the major gap in our knowledge of the field.

A research agenda for economics

The discussion so far indicates two things: first we have a solid understanding of why rational agents cheat by taking drugs, and we can explain, in principle, their reactions to alternative incentive mechanisms designed to abate drug usage; however, secondly, we do not have a very good understanding of the detailed operation of alternative regimes, and we certainly don't know at this stage what constitutes the optimal regime of drug abatement.

To understand these issues from the point of view of economics, a couple of things are needed to be done. First and foremost, more theory is needed – i.e., there is a need to develop a general economic theory of drug usage and drug abatement in sport. To do this, it will be necessary, in the first instance, to understand what it is that the various stakeholders want, which means specifying the utility functions of sportsmen, spectators, peak bodies, the bureaucracy and the media. It will also be necessary to understand how they interact with each other – i.e. to understand what constraints they impose on each other by their conduct. For example, it would be helpful if we better understood the way in which sportsmen respond to different incentive regimes, how spectators regard drug usage, how peak bodies and bureaucracies internalize the attitudes of spectators, how interested the media is in exposing usage to increase sales, and so on. The above arguments have been suggestive of what is required, but have not been more than that.

Once the formal modelling is done, the 'welfare economics' of the theory will then have to be examined. This is to say that the social costs and benefits of each regime will have to be determined under different specifications of parameters so that the optimal abatement regime can be ascertained in each case.

Finally, with the theory in place, it will be necessary to calibrate the models with empirical data so that practical advice might be offered.

This seems like rather a long list of things to be done. However, as remarked upon earlier, economic theory already has available to it the appropriate analytical tools; it merely remains to apply them to the case at hand.

Notes

1 Kahneman and Tversky, 'Prospect Theory: An Analysis of Decision under Risk'.

2 Houlihan, *Dying to Win*. The following is a good sample of the literature: Berentsen, 'The Economics of Doping'; Bird and Wagner, 'Sport as a Common Property Resource'; Haugen, 'The Performance-enhancing Drug Game'; Ehrenberg and Bognanno, 'Do Tournaments have Incentive Effects?'; Kräkel, 'Doping in Contest-like Situations'; Kräkel and Sliwka, 'Risk Taking in Asymmetric Tournaments'; Maennig, 'On the Economics of Doping and Corruption in International Sports'; Preston and Szymanski, 'Cheating in Contests'; Savulescu, Foddy and Clayton, 'Why We Should Allow Performance enhancing Drugs in Sport'; and Szymanski, 'The Economic Design of Sporting Contests'.

3 Milgrom and Roberts, *Economics, Organization and Management*, 367–9.

4 See Berentsen, 'The Economics of Doping'.

5 See Bird and Wagner, 'Sport as a Common Property Resource'.

6 Niskanen, *Bureaucracy and Representative Government.*

7 Brissonneau, 'Deviant Careers: The Case of Cycling'.

8 See Kräkel, 'Doping in Contest-like Situations'.

References

Berentsen, A. 'The Economics of Doping'. *European Journal of Political Economy* 18 (2002): 109–27.

Bird, E.J., and G.G. Wagner. 'Sport as a Common Property Resource'. *Journal of Conflict Resolution* 44, no. 6 (1997): 749–66.

Brissonneau, C. 'Deviant Careers: The Case of Cycling.' WADA Conference *Ethics and Social Science Research in Anti-doping*, Larnaca, Cyprus, April 13–14, 2006.

Ehrenberg, R.G., and M.L. Bognanno. 'Do Tournaments have Incentive Effects?'. *Journal of Political Economy* 98, no. 6 (1990): 1307–24.

Haugen, K. 'The Performance-enhancing Drug Game'. *Journal of Sports Economics* 5, no. 1 (2004): 67–86.

Houlihan, B. *Dying to Win: Doping in Sport and the Development of Anti-doping Policy*. Strasbourg: Council of Europe Press, 2002.

Kahneman, D., and A. Tversky. 'Prospect Theory: An Analysis of Decision under Risk'. *Econometrica* 7, no. 2 (1979): 263–92.

Kräkel, M. 'Doping in Contest-like Situations.' *Governance and the Efficiency of Economic Systems*, Discussion Paper 46, University of Mannheim, Germany, 2006.

Kräkel, M., and D. Sliwka. 'Risk Taking in Asymmetric Tournaments'. *German Economic Review* 5, no. 1 (2004): 103–16.

Maennig, W. 'On the Economics of Doping and Corruption in International Sports'. *Journal of Sports Economics* 3, no. 1 (2002): 61–89.

Milgrom, P., and J. Roberts. *Economics, Organization and Management*. Upper Saddle River, NJ: Prentice Hall, 1992.

Niskanen, W.A. *Bureaucracy and Representative Government*. Chicago, IL: Aldine-Atherton, 1971.

Preston, I., and S. Szymanski. 'Cheating in Contests'. *Oxford Review of Economic Policy* 19, no. 4 (2003): 612–24.

Savulescu, J., B. Foddy, and M. Clayton. 'Why We Should Allow Performance Enhancing Drugs in Sport'. *British Journal of Sports Medicine* 38 (2004): 666–70.

Szymanski, S. 'The Economic Design of Sporting Contests'. *Journal of Economic Literature* 41, no. 4 (2003): 1137–87.

Drugs in sport: the legal issues

Anne Amos and Saul Fridman

Sydney Law School, University of Sydney, Sydney, Australia

The World Anti-Doping Code, the first serious attempt to standardize legal norms internationally, raises a number of difficult legal issues for the legal tools used to implement the Code and whether those tools are consistent with their justifications. For example, the question of an athlete's knowledge or intent to commit a doping infraction is effectively irrelevant in the context of the 'strict liability' standard. We also consider issues connected with the imposition of sanctions, such as proportionality and the enforceability of exclusions from sport as a restraint of trade. In conclusion, we suggest substantial work is needed to develop acceptable legal standards for the 'non-analytical' positive test, where, in the absence of testing positive to a banned substance, circumstantial evidence exists to satisfy a sporting tribunal that an athlete has been involved in a doping infraction. We also suggest much work is needed to establish the strict liability standard, despite its universal acceptance by sporting bodies.

The use of drugs, generally as well as in the context of sporting or other competitive activity, is hardly novel. Most accounts of doping in sport relate episodes going back as far as Greco-Roman times and include anecdotes of the use of various balms, herbs, preparations and animal parts to achieve some real or perceived advantage.[1] Modern attempts to control the use of various substances (usually and originally those thought to provide performance enhancement) dates back to the early part of the twentieth century. In this essay it is our aim to describe the modern legal approach to the regulation of drug use in sport ('doping'). We note that other contributors to this collection are describing philosophical, economic, sociological and psychological approaches to this behaviour.

How the law looks at drugs in sport

The lawyer, as opposed, for example, to the sociologist, takes the problem as a 'given'. That is to say, a policy decision is made to proscribe certain conduct and the lawyer's contribution will usually consist of translating the policy aim into enforceable and rational rules. In the area of doping, as we shall see, this has been particularly problematic. We submit that this is the likely effect of designing rules without proper attention being paid to defining the problem. This may also be the result of *ex post* rationalization. In other words, a decision was taken to proscribe the use of drugs in sport (often without proper consideration of what constitutes a 'drug' for this purpose) followed by the imposition of legal rules.

Assuming away, for the moment, the question of defining 'illicit drugs' in this context, there is also, from the lawyer's perspective, the question of which of many available legal strategies ought to be employed. In relation to so-called recreational drugs generally, most societies have, for better or worse, adopted a strategy of prohibition. This strategy, for the most part, is that used in modern sport. We, as lawyers, seldom question the effectiveness of this strategy, as lawyers tend to assume that prohibition accompanied by sanctions will provide a deterrent effect. We believe that this assumption may not be warranted, and are delighted to be engaged in collaborative research with social scientists that will include consideration of whether this strategy is both effective and appropriate.

Finally, lawyers need to understand questions of procedure and authority: who is to create and enforce the rules that are agreed upon? Whose agreement is necessary? What procedural requirements need to be followed and what will be the effect of failure to adhere to such procedure? When considering such questions in the context of rules that prohibit certain behaviour on pain of sanction, the question of 'rights' inevitably emerges. The legal practitioner, as well as the legal academic, will be particularly concerned to ensure that, in this context, the legitimate rights (whatever they may be) of the athlete are properly protected. Against this consideration is the question of the legitimate interests of the relevant authority.

With the foregoing in mind, this essay:

1. Identifies what the law has done by describing the modern legal framework within which doping activity is regulated;
2. Identifies some of the critical legal issues that have arisen to date and will undoubtedly arise in the future; and,
3. Identifies an agenda for areas of fruitful future legal research.

What the law has done

This essay re-analyses some of the history of drugs in sport from a legal perspective, drawing on the Australian experience from which suggestions for future research in the international context can be drawn. Extrapolating from the Australian context is used as convenient shorthand, as attempting to condense the complexity of international experiences would (and probably should) fill an entire volume in itself. The aim of this historical overview is designed to give readers an insight to, and understanding of, the information used by lawyers and the way lawyers think about drugs in sport, as well as foreshadowing some of the issues that form part of the research agenda.

International doping laws – a primer

The creation of the World Anti-Doping Authority (WADA) in November 1999 was heralded as bringing in a new era in anti-doping, 'a new dimension ... to the fight against doping in sport' because '[with] one historic associative act, sport organizations and governments are now united in their efforts to achieve completely drug free sport'.[2]

While one could trace a reasonably lengthy history of legal and quasi-legal instruments produced to combat doping, we will focus our attention on the legal rules in place since the creation of WADA. In order to understand fully how WADA and the World Anti-Doping Code (WADA Code) were intended to operate, one needs to examine the prior state of anti-doping law.

The pre-WADA situation

Prior to the creation of WADA, anti-doping rules suffered a number of defects, many of which were demonstrated by successful legal challenges to the imposition of sanctions against athletes. In our view, these defects can be summarized under the following headings:

1. The problem of multiple jurisdictions.
2. The problem of 'strict liability'.
3. The problem of inconsistent sanctions.

An understanding of these critical legal issues is essential to developing an understanding of the WADA Code.

1. Multiple jurisdictions

International, national and local sporting activity is organized along a variety of lines. Nationally, different federations (referred to variously as National Federations (NFs) or Sports Governing Bodies (SGBs) control and administer different sports. This issue multiplies when governmental apparatus become involved. The administration of Australian basketball is a good example of the multiple jurisdiction issue given the involvement of a NF, professional league and government. The professional competition is organized by the National Basketball League and other activity, such as selection of a representative team for Olympic and Commonwealth Games, is organized by Basketball Australia. Where there are different organizations with administrative responsibility, there are potentially different rules. To add to this mix, government agencies, both State and Federal, exist for the purpose of promoting sporting activity. Federally, this is the task of the Australian Sports Commission (ASC), which, in the past, promulgated its own specific anti-doping policy. To add to the confusion, the ASC Anti-Doping Policy was, in some respects inconsistent with the model anti-doping policy produced by the International Olympic Committee (IOC) (and adopted for use in this country by the Australian Olympic Committee [AOC]).

Internationally, more confusion reigned, as different rules might be produced by an NF and its international parent (the International Federation [IF]). In one celebrated case an Australian cyclist was able to persuade a Supreme Court Judge in New South Wales to set aside a sanction for a doping violation largely on grounds related to inconsistency between the relevant rules of the NF and IF.[3] Not only was there potential for inconsistency in penalties, but there might be a problem if an athlete was tested by a foreign anti-doping authority.[4]

2. Strict liability

The concept of strict liability relates to the necessity of proving an intention to engage in doping activity as an element of any 'offence'. A strict liability rule does not require such intent to be proved, only that the prohibited activity has been committed. A perennial difficulty in anti-doping efforts is the question of whether 'inadvertent' doping ought to result in the imposition of a sanction. In an age of mandatory testing both in and out of competition, there are circumstances where athletes have tested positive to banned substances after having inadvertently used preparations or medications which, unknown to them, contain traces of substances on the prohibited list.[5] Prior to the development of the WADA Code, there was great inconsistency among the various anti-doping policies on the question of the need to prove an intention to derive an advantage. The various codes had different provisions dealing with permitted therapeutic use as well as different inclusions on the applicable prohibited list for that sport. In addition, some anti-doping policies had provisions setting out 'exceptional circumstances' which might lead to reduction or elimination of any sanction. As we shall see, one of the aims of the WADA Code is to standardize the treatment of so-called 'inadvertent doping' by imposing a tough strict liability standard. The historic operation of the strict liability offence will be considered below in light of the adoption of this approach in the WADA Code.

3. Inconsistent sanctions

At the heart of the WADA Code is not only the concept of strict liability for doping infractions, but also the imposition of standard minimum penalties. As noted above, the pre-WADA Code situation was that each sport had it's own anti-doping rules to which sanctions of varying lengths applied. In the past, athletes have been able to argue successfully that inconsistent penalties among the relevant IFs and NFs provides evidence supporting the proposition that a particular sanction imposed is an unreasonable restraint of trade. Simply put, any time an athlete is subjected to exclusion from their 'profession' for reasons having to do with doping or anything else, the relevant authority must, if called upon to do so, be able to justify the length and scope of any exclusion on the basis of reasonableness.[6] The fact that other sports had imposed lesser sanctions could be used as evidence to show that the length of the particular sanction was not reasonable. This argument will be considered in more detail below.

A cornerstone of the WADA Code is the concept of a fixed minimum two-year sanction for a first 'offence', followed by lifetime exclusion for any subsequent offence. In the debate leading up the creation of WADA and the subsequent development of the WADA Code, this was one of the more contentious issues, as those IFs in sports with highly paid athletes (such as FIFA, the body governing world football) expressed concern about the potential for the body to be sued for damages in cases where the exclusion of an athlete for a minimum period might be found to be in restraint of trade. The WADA Code attempts to deal with this, in part, through provisions setting out 'exceptional circumstances' which allow for reduction in sanctions in special cases. Those responsible for the adoption of the WADA Code argued that it would be appropriate to rely on the Court of Arbitration for Sport (CAS; an arbitral panel given exclusive jurisdiction over doping disputes by the WADA Code; discussed in more detail later in the essay) to develop appropriate legal principles in such cases.

The new era and the WADA Code

This new era began with a number of international doping scandals in 1998: Australian customs officials discovered vials of human growth hormone in the luggage of Chinese swimmers attending the World Swimming Championships; in Germany prosecutions relating to the former state-supported doping of East German athletes continued; Irish Olympic champion swimmer, Michelle de Bruin, was charged with tampering with her urine sample and, in France, customs agents and police uncovered widespread doping in the 1998 Tour de France.[7]

These events, particularly the Tour de France scandal, prompted the IOC Executive Board to hold an international conference on the fight against doping in February 1999.[8] The main result of the conference was the creation of WADA – the first international anti-doping agency. Two years later, in 2003, at a second World Conference, many of the major sports federations and governments agreed to accept the new WADA Code as the universal anti-doping policy for sport. For the first time in history almost all sports and all countries would be subject to the same anti-doping rules. The stated aim of the WADA Code is to 'advance the anti-doping effort through universal harmonization of core anti-doping elements'.[9] The new era in doping has not, however, seen the shedding of all the 'old ways'. Many of the features of past anti-doping policies have been retained. This is due, no doubt, to the fact that the WADA Code was modelled on the Olympic Movement Anti-Doping Code (OMADC) pursuant to the Lausanne Declaration of 1999. The pivotal feature of many of the past anti-doping policies, the use of the strict liability offence, has been maintained in the WADA Code.

Doping offences and the strict liability in the WADA Code

Article 1 of the WADA Code defines doping as 'the occurrence of one or more of the anti-doping rule violations'.

There are a number of Anti-Doping Rule Violations set out in Article 2, the first being the classic strict liability offence:

The following constitute anti-doping rule violations:

2.1 The presence of a Prohibited Substance or its Metabolites or Markers in an Athlete's bodily Specimen.

2.1.1 It is each Athlete's personal duty to ensure that no Prohibited Substance enters his or her body. Athletes are responsible for any Prohibited Substance or its Metabolites or Markers found to be present in their bodily Specimen. Accordingly it is not necessary that intent, fault, negligence or knowing Use on the Athlete's part be demonstrated in order to establish an anti-doping rule violation under Article 2.1.

Other ways in which athletes and associated persons can be found guilty of doping are set out in Articles 2.2 to 2.8. These include 'Use or Attempted Use of a Prohibited Substance or Prohibited Method' (Article 2.2), refusing to provide a sample for testing (Article 2.3), tampering with a sample (Article 2.5), possession (Article 2.6), trafficking (Article 2.7) and ancillary offences (aiding, abetting and so on in Article 2.8).[10] Similar anti-doping rule offences were also contained in the Olympic Movement Anti-Doping Code and the Rules of the International Athletics Associations Federation (IAAF), however, the WADA Code particularises and clarifies these additional offences.[11]

A basic legal definition of a 'strict liability' offence is one in which the prosecution has only to prove the outward or external circumstances of the offence (*actus reus*) without any accompanying mental element (*mens rea*). In relation to the offence of doping, doping authorities need only demonstrate that a prohibited substance has been found in the athlete's bodily specimen, 'it is not necessary that intent, fault, negligence or knowing use on the Athlete's part be demonstrated in order to prove an anti-doping violation'.[12] Ordinarily, the sorts of offences that are designated as strict liability are those toward the lesser end of any scale of moral culpability and in respect of which relatively minor penalties apply.

While the first part of Article 2 clearly defines a 'strict liability offence', the same is not necessarily true of the anti-doping violation, described in Article 2.2, 'the use or attempted use of a Prohibited substance'. At issue here is whether one can in fact 'use' or 'attempt to use' a substance inadvertently. For example Judge Lauri Tarasti of Finland, member of the WADA legal group, was at one time of the view that the expression 'use of' implied a notion of intent.[13] However, the commentary provided with Article 2 of the WADA Code suggests that 'use of' is also strict liability. This is supported by comments by the Court of Arbitration for Sport in the *Mark French v Australian Sports Commission and Cycling Australia*:

> Does the verb 'use' require an interpretation that *mens rea* be an element or does the word 'use' create strict liability? In sporting matters involving anti-doping rules the approach of strict liability has normally been the case.[14]

This approach seems consistent with case law (both pre- and post-WADA Code) where the 'presence of' provision and 'use of' provision appear to have been used almost interchangeably.[15] The difficulty with this position arises from the fact that the WADA Code, and previously the OMADC, contains a provision (Article 2.2.1) which states that the 'success or failure of the use of a prohibited substance' is irrelevant in determining if an athlete has used a prohibited substance. The 'success or failure' provision has been applied in situations where a prohibited substance is detected in the urine specimen of the athlete in the absence of any knowledge or intent. The combination of this statement and interpretation of the 'use of' provision as a strict liability test leads to the situation where a doping sanction can then be applied to an athlete who has neither intended to gain a performance enhancement and in fact has not gained any such enhancement. This is the situation which arose in such cases as *Raducan*, *Baxter*, *Squizzato* and *Puerta*;[16] although none of these athletes had intent to gain a performance enhancement and none of them did actually gain any such enhancement, they were sanctioned for 'doping'. A finding of doping in such circumstances seems at odds with the underlying justifications for anti-doping rules, that is, a desire to maintain the level playing field, since an athlete would not have gained any unfair advantage in these circumstances.

The WADA Code thus overtly adopts the strict liability approach to doping offences. Although fault is not relevant to determination of an offence (and disqualification from the competition is automatic in Article 10.1), the subjective elements of intention or negligence may be taken into account in determining other sanctions (the Period of Ineligibility in Article 10.5). The commentary accompanying this Article in the Code points out that this is the approach taken in Olympic competitions and most other anti-doping codes.

Although many athletes before Tribunals and the Court of Arbitration for Sport have attempted to argue that determination of doping offences does (or should) involve subjective considerations, it has long been the position that most anti-doping policies incorporate the strict liability test. Not only have Tribunals accepted this approach, but also the English High Court of Justice and the Court of Arbitration for Sport in numerous cases.[17]

The history of anti-doping cases show that the strict liability rule has been applied in a number of cases even where reasonable 'excuses' appeared to exist. Below is a list of circumstances in which the rule has been applied in the past:

- An athlete was given a Digesic headache pill by her coach. There was no evidence that the tablet would enhance the performance of the athlete.[18]
- An athlete was inadvertently given one tablet of Effortil by her coach with her food and drink at a major competition where she had no control over what she was eating. There was no evidence that this substance would enhance the performance of the athlete.[19]
- An athlete was given a painkiller by the coach after sustaining an injury in training. The coach had checked the name of the product but not the ingredients of the medication in the list of prohibited substances. The whole team was disqualified.[20]
- A 16-year-old athlete was given cold medication by her team doctor before an Olympic event which contained pseudoephedrine. There was no evidence to suggest that this tablet would have enhanced her performance. The athlete was stripped of her gold medal.[21]
- An athlete was competing in a foreign country and purchased what appeared to be the same product (a Vicks inhaler) as he regularly used at home. He did not read the ingredients. His Olympic bronze medal was removed.[22]

So consistent is the approach of the Court of Arbitration for Sport to the strict liability issue in such cases that Straubel regarded it as applying the strict liability rule 'almost regardless of the rules being applied' (that is, regardless of which sporting body's doping policy was being applied).[23] The past jurisprudence of the court in this regard seems to be reflected in the approach of the WADA Code in subjective elements are to be taken into account only in determining the ongoing sanction but not the actual offence of doping.[24]

As can be seen from the cases illustrated above, there appears to be situations where the imposition of the strict liability rule produces a result that is undeniably harsh to the athlete concerned. In addition to those situations outlined above (referred to as 'inadvertent doping') cases of 'innocent doping' such as the administration of banned substances against the athletes will, a competitor or support person deceitfully placing a banned substance in the food or drink of an athlete or passive inhalation of cannabis smoke have been identified as further circumstances where the rule would produce injustice.[25] It is this aspect of anti-doping regulation that has been the source of most criticism.

Buti and Fridman argue that, given the nature of the sanctions imposed, the defence of honest and reasonable mistake, which is available in criminal cases of strict liability such as *He Kaw Teh v The Queen* should also be available in doping cases.[26] It is submitted that this is particularly the case when the list of prohibited substances is not exhaustive. For example, UK athletes Saxton and Davies and Alain Baxter were disciplined for the use of an unlisted substance because it was held to be a 'related substance'.[27] As Straubel rightly points out, as the definition of the doping offence stands, in the absence of any other defence, an athlete would have to show that there has been some flaw in the testing process in order to overcome the strict liability rule.[28]

Given the problems with the strict liability rule, the question needs to be asked, why has it been adopted in the WADA Code?

The justification for the strict liability offence in the WADC

Fortunately we do not have to use guesswork to assess the justification behind the use of the strict liability offence in the WADC. The reasons for its inclusion are provided in the comment to the strict liability offence, Article 2.1.1. The rationale is stated in the words of the CAS in *Q v International Shooting Union*:

> It is true that a strict liability test is likely in some sense to be unfair in an individual case, such as that of Q, where the Athlete may have taken medication as the result of mislabelling or faulty advice for which he or she is not responsible – particularly in the circumstances of sudden illness in a foreign country. But it is also in some sense 'unfair' for an Athlete to get food poisoning on the eve of an important competition. Yet in neither case will the rules of the competition be altered to undo the unfairness. Just as the competition will not be postponed to await the Athlete's recovery, so the prohibition on banned substances will not be lifted in recognition of its accidental absorption. The vicissitudes of competition, like those of life generally, may create many types of unfairness, whether by accident or the negligence of unaccountable Persons, which the law cannot repair.
>
> Furthermore, it appears to be a laudable policy objective not to repair an accidental unfairness by creating an intentional unfairness to the whole body of other competitors. This is what would happen if banned performance-enhancing substances were tolerated when absorbed inadvertently. Moreover, it is likely that even intentional abuse would in many cases escape sanction for lack of proof of guilty intent. And it is certain that a requirement of intent would invite costly litigation that may well cripple federations – particularly those run on modest budgets – in their fight against doping.[29]

Two main arguments are put forward here. Firstly it is thought that by allowing a competitor to compete with a doping substance in their system, it is creating unfairness for the rest of the cohort of competitors. This is undoubtedly a reference to the level playing field argument that is so prominent in discussions relating to the aims of anti-doping rules. The logic of the court is that even though an athlete may not have intended to enhance their performance, the mere presence of a banned substance would result in unfairness to the other competitors, since they had to compete against an athlete with a prohibited substance in their system.

This kind of reasoning is evident in comments made by the CAS panel in *C v FINA*:

> It would indeed be shocking to include in a ranking an athlete who had not competed using the same means as his opponents for whatever reasons. 'The result of the event has indeed been objectively vitiated and, consequently, the intention of the author is irrelevant.'[30]

Similar attitudes have been expressed by academic commentators:

> Further, there can be no objection in principle from disqualifying anyone who has won a race with the aid of drugs, even though he, she or it was entirely innocent in the matter. The fact remains that the advantage has been gained – and, in objective terms, unfairly.[31]

How far this level playing field argument accurately reflects the reality of inadvertent doping is questionable, particularly in light of the fact that there are substances on the WADA Code *Prohibited List* which do not enhance performance in all sports and some probably do not enhance performance in any sport.[32]

The second rationale presented is the need for effective enforcement of the anti-doping rules. It is argued that the strict liability offence is an essential tool in effective enforcement since doping authorities would not have the resources to uncover evidence of intent on the part of the doping athlete; in order to actually have an effective anti-doping regime, the strict liability offence must be maintained. This argument appears to be the basis on which Rigozzi, Kaufmann-Kohler and Malinverni[33] find that the strict liability rule is justified and also why courts have found that the restraint of trade imposed by such a rule is reasonable. Again, this argument may become less persuasive in the future as enforcement of anti-doping policies increasingly comes under the jurisdiction of state-funded investigation bodies, either general law enforcement personnel of specifically trained and resourced anti-doping bodies, rather than sporting federations.

It should be noted here that the CAS admits that in some individual cases the strict liability offence will result in unfairness for the athlete involved. Here the court is accepting that some of the criticisms of the strict liability rule in inadvertent doping situations are justified and inherent in a strict liability system. However, the court, like many other bodies and commentators, accept that any unfairness to the individual is outweighed by considerations in the authority's interests.

Specified substances and exceptional circumstances

In recognition of the problems inherent in the strict liability rule the WADA Code also includes provisions designed to ameliorate the harshness of the approach. These are the specified substances (Article 10.3) and exceptional circumstances provisions (Article 10.5). As well as these provisions there have been changes to the Prohibited List, particularly removal of pseudoephedrine, which will deal with a number of inadvertent doping problems.[34]

Under Article 10.3, the applicable Ineligibility Period will be reduced if the athlete is able to show that use of a specified substance was not intended to enhance performance. A specified substance is a prohibited substance which has been specifically identified on the Prohibited List, being substances 'particularly susceptible to unintentional anti-doping rule violations because of their general availability in medicinal products or which are less likely to be successfully abused as doping agents'. Examples of specified substances include: glucocorticosteroids, alcohol, beta-blockers, cannabinoids, ephedrine and a number of other stimulants.

If the athlete successfully argues that they did not intend to enhance sport performance then the ineligibility period can be reduced to a minimum of a warning and reprimand and maximum of one year suspension for a first offence while a second offence attracts a two year suspension. Life ineligibility will only apply after a third offence under this section.

Under Article 10.5 there is also opportunity for the doping panel to take into account the level of fault of the athlete in determining the length of the Ineligibility Period. The Ineligibility Period, i.e. the period of suspension after the relevant competition, can be either eliminated or reduced due to exceptional circumstances under this article. If the athlete is able to show that there was no fault or negligence on their part and can establish how the prohibited substance came to be in their system then the Ineligibility Period can be eliminated. The commentary to Article 10.5.2 gives an example of where this section may apply; in the case where 'despite all due care he or she was sabotaged by a competitor'. Examples of where the Ineligibility Period *will not* be reduced are also provided: sabotage by someone within the athlete's entourage, administration by the athlete's physician without the athlete's knowledge and mislabelled or contaminated supplements.

If the athlete is unable to meet the high standard of 'no fault or negligence' then Article 10.5.2, 'no significant fault or negligence', may be relevant. According to the commentary, some of the situations listed above, although not eliminating the Ineligibility Period under Article 10.5.1, might lead to a reduction under Article 10.5.2. If the athlete can show that there was no significant fault on their part and can establish how the prohibited substance came to be in their system, then the Ineligibility Period may be reduced by up to half the applicable period (Article 10.2 sets out these periods as two years for a first offence and life for a second offence).

Although these provisions do explicitly provide for reduction of the mandatory sanctions, even successful cases under these provisions lead to automatic disqualification. Furthermore it has been difficult for athletes to successfully bring cases under the exceptional circumstances provisions; the tests for application of the sections, set out in Definition section in Appendix 1 of the Code, are quite onerous.[35] Only one athlete has so far had their Ineligibility Period terminated under the new Code.[36] A number of other athletes have had their Ineligibility Period reduced under the 'no significant fault or negligence' provisions. Notwithstanding this, the fact that athletes have been punished for doping in situations where they appear to have very little control (such as accidentally ingesting colourless, odourless, tasteless medications from drinking from the same glass as their wife) still appears quite harsh.

Therefore, despite some 'softening' of the strict liability offence in the WADA Code, the future under the new Code will undoubtedly reveal more difficult inadvertent doping cases just as there was under the predecessors to the Code.

Proof of Doping

Article 3 of the WADA Code deals with the way in which an anti-doping rule violation can be proved or disproved.

Pursuant to the strict liability approach and the anti-doping cases up to this point,[37] a National Anti-Doping Organisation (NADO) must prove that an anti-doping violation has occurred. In Article 3.2.1 of the WADA Code, the onus of proof appears to shift to the athlete once the organization adduces evidence of a positive drug test from a WADA-Accredited Laboratory. If the athlete can rebut the presumption that the international standard for testing has been complied with, the NADO then has to show that the departure did not cause the positive drug result.[38]

Straubel is critical of this presumption in favour of adherence to the correct procedure as it effectively shifts the burden of proof to the athlete to prove their innocence.[39] To prove that the international standard was not adhered to would seem difficult given that the athlete is not present at the testing and evidence must be attained from the laboratory (which may have a vested interest in defending its procedures). Straubel's criticism seems particularly relevant to cases such as Modahl where appropriate documentation regarding the chain of custody was not provided in the first instance. It was later discovered that the samples had been stored unrefrigerated for two days.[40] Despite these concerns, the WADA Code has incorporated the presumption in favour of the anti-doping organization. Perhaps successful challenges to the testing procedures, such as Vinnicombe's case,[41] have convinced the drafters of the Code that the presumption is not unreasonable.

Article 3.1 sets the standard of proof as somewhere between civil and criminal standards of proof, that is 'to the comfortable satisfaction of the hearing body bearing in mind the seriousness of the allegations'. This standard is consistent with a number of tribunal decisions and the standard which has developed in the case law of the CAS.[42]

Right to a fair hearing

Recognition of a right to a fair hearing is expressed in Article 8. Although it is clear that the hearing process of the Anti-Doping Organisation still stands, the WADA Code sets out principles which that hearing process must abide by. These include:

- A timely hearing
- Fair and impartial hearing body
- The right to be represented by counsel at the person's own expense
- The right to be fairly and timely informed of the asserted anti-doping rule violation
- The right to respond to the asserted anti-doping rule violation
- The right of each party to present evidence, including the right to call and question witnesses (subject to the hearing body's discretion to accept testimony by telephone or written submissions)
- The Person's right to an interpreter at the hearing, with the hearing body to determine the identity, and responsibility for the cost, of the interpreter; and
- A timely, written, reasoned decision.

The principles set out in the Code reflect a desire to overcome a number of problems related to due process or natural justice which have been identified by numerous authors in anti-doping cases to date.

One aspect of anti-doping cases which has been identified as potentially involving a breach of procedural fairness is where an athlete was not notified of any known offence. The case usually mentioned in this regard is that of Saxton and Davies where two athletes were suspended from the Olympic Games and sent home after testing positive to Clenbuterol without a hearing. Clenbuterol was not on the applicable Prohibited List until after this decision had been made.[43] Although the Court of Arbitration for Sport accepted in other cases that there is a right to be heard,[44] it appears from these cases that this has not been applied universally by sporting tribunals.

It has also been suggested that on a number of occasions anti-doping tribunals have breached the rules of natural justice through actual bias or the appearance of bias.[45] Cases identified as involving this problem include *Modahl v The British Athletic Federation Ltd* where a spokesman of the Federation deciding her case publicly expressed his opinion as to her guilt;[46] *Reynolds v IAAF US District Court, Sth District of Ohio* where the court recognized the IAAF was biased and Merlene Ottey where the Federation was acting as decision maker and also representing the defendant.[47]

It is interesting to note that the WADA Code establishes both the right to have counsel present and the right to have a timely, written, reasoned decision provided, both of which have been raised as issues of natural justice in doping cases.[48] Codifying the principles of a fair and impartial hearing body is an attempt to overcome these problems.

One aspect of doping cases which has attracted criticism has not been addressed by the WADA Code. Suspension by the relevant federation can be imposed on the athlete before the holding of the hearing.[49] Blair argues that this, in itself, is not a violation of the principles of natural justice but that *public announcement* of a positive drug test prior to a hearing may be.[50] It appears that both practices could continue under the WADA Code as Article 7.5 allows a provisional suspension once the athlete has been notified of the positive drug test but before the hearing, while Article 14.2 allows public disclosure after notification but presumably before the hearing.[51]

Therapeutic use exemption

In cases where athletes need to use medications which contain prohibited substances a therapeutic use exemption is available with medical certification. Article 4.4 of the WADA Code and the *International Standard for Therapeutic Use Exemptions* (TUE) sets a 21-day cut off for the application for a Therapeutic Use Exemption. Applications after this time will only be allowed in limited cases (emergency treatment and unforeseen circumstances). It appears that under the WADA Code there is little scope for the flexible approach taken by the CAS in the case of *L v FINA*.[52] There the court determined that no doping offence should be recorded when an athlete failed to apply for a TUE for his asthma medication because the evidence showed that it was well known by officials that he used this particular medication on medical authority. It would appear that the drafters of the WADA Code have preferred the approach of recording an offence and a subsequent reduction in the sanction by way of Article 10.5 (elimination or reduction of period of ineligibility based on exceptional circumstances). It may be difficult for athletes to use these provisions particularly in acute medical situations suggesting that such a strategy would result in a number of athletes with legitimate medical problems being sanctioned for doping offences. Perhaps this is to deter athletes from making the type of oversight involved in L's case.

Sanctions

The pre-Code position was that sporting organizations determined the applicable sanctions for the offence, allowing for variation in sanctions between sports. As noted above the Code has introduced universally applicable sanctions.

Sanctions for violations are set forth in Articles 9 and 10 of the Code. Disqualification from the relevant competition is automatic once a violation has occurred. Additional sanctions for doping offences, the Ineligibility Period, are suspension for two years for the first offence and a lifetime ban for a second. Article 10.5 allows exceptional circumstances to be taken into account in reducing the additional sanction (discussed above). The commentary to these Articles notes that although, as noted above, the mandatory two year/life time sanctions are some of the most controversial aspects of anti-doping policy (as the same sanction may have a more significant impact on some sports than others), the World Conference on Doping in Sport came to the consensus that the Olympic rules should be followed.

As noted above Australian commentators have given some attention to the possibility that mandatory sanctions, coupled with strict liability offences, could be challenged as an unreasonable restraint of trade.[53] Although the English Court in *Gasser v Stinson* considered that the principle could be applied to anti-doping cases, it accepted that the restraint was not unreasonable given the objectives of anti-doping programmes.[54] Two Australian cases have invoked the principle, one successfully.[55] Buti and Fridman argue that the legitimate public interest of protecting the athlete's right to compete and the interests of the sporting body being protected need to be weighed against the public interest in banning 'drug cheats'.[56] They suggest that the penalties for doping offences could be seen as unreasonable restraints of trade given the invasion of privacy, the possible application of the criminal law and the extent to which consent to drug testing is not truly voluntary. Such an argument may be even more likely with the acceptance of the sanctions set out in the WADA Code, since there appears little opportunity to relate the sanction to the usual length of an athlete's career in a particular sport.[57] This suggests that problems identified with sanctions in the past are set to become more of an issue under the new Code.

The role of the Court of Arbitration for Sport (CAS)

Article 13.2.1 nominates the CAS as the exclusive forum for appeals involving international-level athletes. Appeals concerning domestic-level athletes are dealt with in Article 13.2.2, and are to be dealt with according to the rules of the NADO. In most cases, these appeals are either to CAS or a panel of arbitrators established under the relevant rules.

In either case, the preferred means of disposing of appeals is by arbitration. Notably, the principal advantage of arbitration (aside from possible savings in cost and time) is that the appeal will be decided by a panel of experts. The CAS has established itself over the years as the leading source of reasoned analysis of anti-doping rules.

For the present, we note that arbitration remains, like litigation in the civil courts, an adversarial model of dispute resolution. That is to say, the matter proceeds on the basis of each party presenting its case before a panel of referees for their determination. To be sure, in many cases (including the CAS) the rules of evidence and procedure can be relaxed. Indeed, an advantage of the CAS is its willingness to convene panels quickly and in a variety of locations. Nonetheless, as with drug policy generally, there are those who suggest that a less adversarial model of dispute resolution, such as mediation or conciliation, would be more appropriate. For the present, suffice it to say that it is hard to imagine mediation being successful in an environment where minimum sanctions are imposed. An athlete would have little incentive (beyond that already offered in Article 10.5 dealing with exceptional circumstances) to cooperate. Clearly this is an area where further research would be helpful.

The impact of the WADA Code

Of course it is too early to make convincing claims about the effectiveness of the WADA Code. At the time of writing this article (2006–07), the Code has only been in existence for about four years and fully applied only in the two most recent Olympic Games (Athens 2004 and Torino 2006). It is clear that the careful drafting of Article 2 (incorporating the strict liability principle) and the inclusion of the specified substances and exceptional circumstances provisions aim to clarify some of the issues that have arisen in previous legal proceedings. Nonetheless, as substances become harder and harder to detect, authorities (as we are already starting to see) are increasingly relying on what are becoming known as 'non-analytical positives'.[58] These cases involve assertions that the athlete is 'in possession' of banned substances or is 'involved in' a contravention and rely on the provisions of Articles 2.2–2.8.[59] As we have suggested above, some legal issues remain to be determined, such as the extent to which it is possible, for purposes of proof of a doping event, to possess a substance without knowing of its presence. There will also, no doubt, be issues relating to the sufficiency of evidence as there are in all cases built of circumstantial evidence. As experience in the BALCO (Bay Area Laboratory Co-operative) cases in the United States have shown, this will be a particular difficulty in the 'court' of public opinion when the public are so used to a system of doping rules which relies almost exclusively on scientific proof of doping via urine or blood tests.[60]

Despite public suspicion of the non-analytical positive, many see them as an effective new 'tool' for anti-doping enforcement.[61] Whether such cases are likely to displace drug testing and the strict liability approach is somewhat doubtful though. Difficulties with gathering sufficient evidence and the expense of both prosecuting and defending such cases are two of the factors which may weigh against the use of the non-analytical positive case in the future.[62] Certainly so far under the WADA Code the cases suggest that strict liability and drug testing will continue to be of importance in anti-doping efforts for some time to come.

What the law needs to know

As we have previously suggested, research into doping law has been largely descriptive, focusing on describing the present system of rules and the way in which they work (at least up to when this essay was written). As legal practitioners, we tend to focus on how to do our job best: advising an athlete who is seeking to avoid falling foul of the rules, prosecuting a case on behalf of the authority or defending an athlete against a charge of doping. Thus to this point legal research into doping in sport has focused on the mechanisms of the law. This kind of research is by no means complete, and indeed doping law is a particularly challenging area for everyday lawyers, not least due to the difficulties involved in accessing previous doping case law. This means that doping cases are generally left to a very few specialists.

In this brief review of the key legal issues, one can see that there is still some work to be done to translate the philosophical and policy aims of anti-doping programmes into workable legal rules. Along with other social scientists, we need to explore the best means of effecting this translation. This might be an area for collaboration between lawyers and political scientists or public administration experts.[63]

Furthermore, a particular lack in the area of research in doping law are well researched answers to the more fundamental questions. These questions largely relate to programme evaluation and the attempt to measure the effectiveness of whether the anti-doping effort is achieving its ideological goals. Direct questions that we as lawyers, members of the public, and sports fans want answers to, include:

- Is this system working?
- Is it fair?
- Is there a better way?
- Are we achieving what we want to achieve?
- Are we even achieving what we think we are achieving in doping law?

All these questions remain largely unanswered. Some, of course are presently unanswerable. Due to the clandestine nature of drug use in sport it is difficult to tell the prevalence of drug use[64] and, since we have had no other regulatory system of doping to compare with, whether the prohibitionist approach has been more effective than other approaches. We have therefore outlined below some areas of possible research which may answer some of the more *answerable* questions about doping law.

A research agenda for the law

The three areas of research presented below appear to be ones which are both achievable and useful in answering some of the questions which have not been answered to this point in time. They may help us to get a more accurate picture of the effect of doping law and thus help us evaluate the extent to which our anti-doping system is fulfilling its role and goals.

Strict liability

The first issue of importance is the strict liability rule. Anecdotal evidence from case law suggests that there are still cases where athletes, inadvertently or otherwise, have fallen foul of the strict liability rules in circumstances where there is neither risk to health nor any realistic chance of obtaining a performance-enhancing effect. And, of course, the decided CAS arbitrations are only a small part of the entire picture. At a blunt level, more work needs to be done to test the true effectiveness of the current WADA Code model. This might include an examination of whether its 'exceptional circumstances' provisions are sufficient to deal with the deserving cases. Indeed, more work needs to be done to define what exactly those 'deserving cases' are.

Of first importance appears to be to answer the question of whether the current system, that is the total prohibition/strict liability system, actually deters the use of drugs in sport. As noted above, it would appear practically impossible to determine whether the strict liability rule deters intentional drug users in sport. It is almost universally accepted that the number of positive doping tests is by no means a good indicator of the number of athletes using drugs, mostly because of the inadequacies of drug testing to keep up with developments in doping agents.[65] And thus the corollary is also true: lack of positive drug tests does not indicate the number of 'clean' athletes. It is also highly unlikely that those using drugs with intention would admit, even anonymously, that they are using prohibited substances.[66] It appears therefore almost impossible to examine the deterrent effect of the strict liability rule on intentional drug users.

However, one of the proposed effects of the strict liability rule will be to make athletes more careful of what they ingest. It is argued that by making the athlete absolutely responsible for anything found in their bodies it will increase their level of vigilance regarding prohibited substances in general and therefore make the use of doping substances less likely.[67] It would be possible to examine this aspect of the effect of the strict liability rule by way of some well modelled interviews which would seek to examine what precautions athletes take to avoid prohibited substances; whether the athlete is willing to trust other people (other athletes, doctors, managers, coaches etc.) regarding whether a substance in prohibited; how often they would use doping advisory services; whether they take any supplements (which have often led to inadvertent positives) and so on. All these questions may give us some indicator of whether the current system is affecting athletes' behaviour. Research into the role of support staff and the approach taken by regulators[68] to them would also be helpful.

Alternatives to strict liability

The second area of research which appears to be both possible and useful would focus on the provisions of the WADA Code which seek to ameliorate the recognized harshness of the strict liability rule. There are a number of such provisions outlined above, including the 'exceptional circumstances' provisions, the 'specified substances' provisions and the 'therapeutic use exemptions'. Similar interviews and surveys of athletes and support personnel as to the effectiveness of these provisions could give some indicator of how they work 'on the ground'. For instance, sports doctors may be able to give insight into the kind of circumstances in which they are able to use the therapeutic use exemptions and circumstances where they are not able to. Athletes may be able to reveal how often they are unable to use certain medications which they need. Research of case law after the provisions came into effect will also show some instances of the way in which these provisions work in real life situations. Results of this research might be helpful in evaluating the appropriateness of the adversarial dispute resolution model presently in use.

Harmonisation: the effect of sanctions across sports and athletes

The final area of research which could answer some of these fundamental questions relates to the imposition of universal sanctions. What has been of most concern in this regard has been the differential effect that the same sanction may have on athletes from different sports, athletes in some sports having a much longer career than others. It has been argued that imposing the same sanction on two athletes from different sports could virtually end the career of one while amounting to no more that an extended vacation in the career of the other.[69] One area of potential research would be to investigate the careers of athletes who have been affected by the doping rules to see how the imposition of various sanctions has affected their career. Questions such as whether they returned to competition, how long they continued to compete, how the sanction affected them financially and whether they were able to return to the same level as they previously had achieved would all give some indictor of the effect of the sanction. Such data could then be examined to see whether there were any particular patterns with regard to the various sports; did gymnasts who were sanctioned for doping routinely drop out of their sport for instance?

These kinds of research questions might give us some idea of whether we are doing what we think we are doing in our anti-doping programmes. The answers may help to shape such programmes in the future.[70]

Notes

1 Verroken, 'Drug Use and Abuse in Sport'.

2 Juan Antonio Samaranch, 'Minutes of the Inaugural Meeting of the Board of the World Anti-Doping Authority (WADA)', January 13, 2000, Olympic House, Lausanne. http://www.wada-ama.org/rtecontent/document/130100-ENG.pdf; Richard Pound, 'Message from the Chairman', WADA. http://www.wada-ama.org/en/dynamic.ch2?pageCategory_id=1.

3 *Robertson v Australian Professional Cycling Council Inc.* In Robertson's case, the doctrine of restraint of trade (discussed later in this essay) was applied to strike the sanction as unreasonable.

4 In *Vinnicombe v Australian Sports Drug Agency,* Martin Vinnicombe, an Australian cyclist, was tested by the Canadian Anti-Doping Authority while competing at an event in the US. Vinnicombe successfully challenged sanctions imposed for testing positive to stanozolol in part on the basis that the Canadian authorities were not authorized to perform tests under the relevant Australian legislation and therefore he could not be taken to have returned a positive test result within the meaning of the relevant rules.

5 There are a number of cases, for example, involving ephedrine and pseudo-ephedrine, both of which are commonly found in many cold medications. In *Baxter v IOC* the athlete used an over-the-counter medication without knowing that the product available in the US (sold under the same brand name as that which he used in the UK) contained a banned stimulant. Neither the athlete's 'innocence' nor the fact that the substance in question provided arguably no performance enhancement was relevant to the question of whether the athlete was to be excluded for having contravened the relevant doping policy.

6 Based on *Nordenfelt v Maxim Nordenfelt Guns and Ammunition Co Ltd*, the basic law in this area has been unchanged for over a century and requires the party defending the sanction to establish that the sanction is reasonable in the interests of both the parties (i.e. that it does not exceed what is necessary to protect the legitimate interests of the association) and the public (i.e. that the resulting exclusion is not so broad as to offend 'public policy').

7 Ferstle, 'Evolution and Politics of Drug Testing', 275–6.

8 Judge Kéba Mbaye, 'Report of the Working Group on the Legal and Political Aspects of Doping', 1.

9 'World Anti-Doping Code'. www.wada-ama.org/rtecontent/document/code_v3.pdf, 2003, 1.

10 Important to note here is that these ancillary provisions quite clearly extend the reach of the WADA Code to support staff (trainers, dieticians, coaches, managers and any other person involved with the athlete).

11 The *Olympic Movement Anti-Doping Code (OMAC),* Chapter II, Article 2, 'the use of an expedient' and Article 1, 'Recommending, proposing, authorizing', current as at February 1999; see also Beloff, 'Drugs, Law and Versapaks'.

12 'World Anti-Doping Code', Article 2.1.1.

13 See Beloff, 'Drugs, Law and Versapaks', 44. See also Opie, 'Legal Regimes for the Control of Performance-enhancing Drugs in Sport', 347, who also argues that 'uses or takes advantage of' is likely to involve intent on the part of the athlete.

14 *French v Australian Sports Commission and Cycling Australia*, 11.

15 See *Raducan v International Olympic Committee*, and *Baxter v IOC.*

16 See *Raducan v International Olympic Committee*, *Baxter v IOC*, *Squizzato v FINA* and *Puerta v ITF.*

17 See for example '*ATP v Ulihrach* – Decision of the ATP Tour Anti-Doping Tribunal on the Appeal of Bohdan Ulihrach', April 22, 2003. www.atptennis.com/insideATP, 36; and *Gasser v Stinson and Holt.*

18 *V v FINA*; Scott Volkers was Samantha Riley's coach and was disciplined for his involvement in Riley's inadvertent use of a prohibited substance.

19 *C v FINA.*

20 *National Wheelchair Basketball v International Paralympic Committee.*

21 *Raducan v International Olympic Committee.*

22 *Baxter v IOC.*

23 Straubel, 'Doping Due Process', 150.

24 Oschutz, 'Harmonization of Anti-Doping Code through Arbitration', 698, terms this 'additional sanctions' because the acceptance of strict liability means automatic disqualification from the competition in which the positive test was conducted. See *C v FINA* and *V v FINA* for examples of where the court took this approach.

25 Opie, 'Legal Regimes for the Control of Performance-enhancing Drugs in Sport', 344, discusses the implications for food or drink, and Buti and Fridman, *Drugs, Sport and the Law*, 114, discuss passive inhalation of cannabis.

26 Buti and Fridman, 'Drug Testing in Sport', 153; *He Kaw Teh v The Queen.*

27 For discussion on Saxton and Davies see Grayson, 'Drugs, Sport and the Olympics', 1171, and Buti and Fridman, 'The Intersection of Law and Policy', 494. A 'related substance' is defined by the IOC in *Baxter v IOC.* See also J. Magnay, 'White Drug Scandal Rocks US Team'. *Sydney Morning Herald*, June 20, 2003, Sports section, 34, for a similar case.

28 See Straubel, 'Doping Due Process', 543. Exceptions to this statement would include challenges to due process or some other exceptional occurrence such as that which arose in the case of tennis play Bohdan

Ulihrach, where ATP staff administered substances which contained a banned substance. Although technically a doping offence had still occurred the charges were dropped in Ulihrach's case. World Anti-Doping Agency, 'WADA Report on ATP Doping Cases' (2004). http://www.wada-ama.org/rtecontent/document/wada_atp_report.pdf, 1.

29 *Q v International Shooting Union*, 193.

30 Louis Dalléves, as cited in *C v FINA*, 220.

31 See Beloff, 'Drugs, Law and Versapaks', 45.

32 The case of the cricketer, Shane Warne, is a good example of a case where a prohibited substance was taken inadvertently which would have had no performance-enhancing effect on the particular sport involved, as discussed on the ABC Anti-Doping Panel, *Decision: Shane Warne*. http://www.abc.net.au/mediawatch/documents/acb_findings_warne.pdf. Melethil, 'Making the WADA Prohibited List: Show Me The Data', 75 notes that cannabinoids are the primary example here.

33 Rigozzi, Kaufman-Kohler and Malinverni, 'Doping and the Fundamental Rights of Athletes', 39.

34 This substance, commonly found in cold and hay fever medications, has been responsible for a number of inadvertent doping cases in the past.

35 See McLaren, 'CAS Doping Jurisprudence', 32; Foschi, 'A Constant Battle', 457, and Amos, 'Inadvertent Doping and the WADA Code', for more detailed discussion.

36 See the case of Oliferenko in 'IOC Laments 'Mistake by Doctor' Strips Rowing Medals'. http://www.usatoday.com/sports/olympics/athens/boat/2004-08-26-doping-ukraine_x.htm.

37 See comments by Oschutz, 'Harmonization of Anti-Doping Code through Arbitration', 701, that the Court of Arbitration for Sport has shown inconsistency in distinguishing between the strict liability offence and the presumption of guilt.

38 Article 3.2.2 states that departures that don't cause an adverse finding won't invalidate the rules. This clarifies a previously confused position regarding the rebuttable presumption of guilt. See Oschutz, 'Doping Cases before the CAS and the World Anti-Doping Code', 25.

39 See Straubel, 'Doping Due Process', 531 and 548.

40 See Grayson, 'Drugs, Sport and the Olympics'; Buti and Fridman, *Drugs, Sport and the Law*, 106.

41 See *Vinnicombe v Australian Sports Drug Agency*.

42 For the US Track and Field Tribunal as an example, see Straubel, 'Doping Due Process', 536. Fitzgerald, 'The Court of Arbitration for Sport; Dealing with Doping and Due Process during the Olympics', 235. See *B v FINA*, CAS 98/211 at paragraph 25 in Reeb, *Recueil des sentences du TAS Digest of CAS Awards II*, 255, for an articulation of this standard by the CAS. The standard of proof is likely similar to that applied by the High Court in *Briginshaw v Briginshaw*, where, in the application of a civil standard of proof, the nature and consequence of the facts to be proved are appropriate considerations. As Dixon, J., in that case at 362–3 put it 'When, in a civil proceeding, a question arises whether a crime has been committed, the standard of persuasion is, according to the better opinion, the same as upon other civil issues ... But, consistently with this opinion, weight is given to the presumption of innocence and exactness of proof is required'.

43 Kavanagh, 'The Doping Cases and the Need for the International Court of Arbitration for Sport (CAS)', 725.

44 See *Q v International Shooting Union*, 203, for example.

45 Actual bias is discussed by Hatch, 'On Your Marks, Get Set, Stop!', 557, and the appearance of bias by Blair, 'Procedural Fairness in Doping Disputes', 888–9.

46 *Modahl v The British Athletic Federation Ltd.*

47 See Blair, 'Procedural Fairness in Doping Disputes', 890.

48 See Buti and Fridman, 'Drug Testing in Sport', 161.

49 See Straubel, 'Doping Due Process', 548, and Hatch, 'On Your Marks, Get Set, Stop!', 565, for the American context.

50 See Blair, 'Procedural Fairness in Doping Disputes', 887. Although not officially sanctioned announcements, similar damage has no doubt been done in situations where information about doping results have been leaked by the media. Two recent high profile 'victims' of such leaking are Lance Armstrong and Ian Thorpe. Both cases illustrate the perceived damage that such information being made public can cause.

51 That is, once WADA Code, Article 7.1 and 7.2 have been complied with.

52 *L v FINA*.

53 See Buti and Fridman, *Drugs, Sport and the Law*, 126, and Opie 'Legal Regimes for the Control of Performance-enhancing Drugs in Sport', 352.

54 See *Gasser v Stinson and Holt*.

55 *Pate and Hall v Australian Professional Cycling Council Incorporated* and *Robertson v Australian Professional Cycling Council Inc.*

56 See Buti and Fridman, *Drugs, Sport and the Law*, 164ff.
57 Houlihan, *Dying to* Win, 176.
58 The BALCO case is just one example of a growing tendency for anti-doping agencies increasingly relying evidence other than positive drug tests to prove doping violations. Indeed the Australian Sports Anti-Doping Agency (ASADA) has made this an explicit strategy to deal with the new non-detectable substances. See the ASADA annual report, 2005/2006. http://www.asada.gov.au/resources/reports/current/ar06/_docs/asda_ar_2005_06.pdf, 2. This does not mean, however that drug testing and the strict liability rule is set to become relics of the past. Drug testing is still a 'core function' of ASADA.
59 *French v ASC and Cycling Australia* for instance. See also United States Anti-Doping Agency, 'Former World Champion Collins Receives Eight-year Suspension for Participation in BALCO Drug Conspiracy', and Mark Fainaru-Wada and Lance Williams, 'Montgomery Banned for Doping. World record Expunged; Gaines also Banned'. *San Francisco Chronicles*, December 14, 2005. http://www.sfgate.com/cgi-bin/article.cgi?f=/c/a/2005/12/14/SPG8BG7Q681.
60 See Sally Jenkins, 'This Agency Lacks the Inside Dope'. *The Washington Post*, May 17, 2004. http://www.washingtonpost.com/wp-dyn/articles/A31738-2004May16.html. Jenkins, 'This is Wrong: USADA has Athletes Guilty Until Proven Guilty'. *The Washington Post*, May 20, 2004. http://www.journalnow.com; and Tim Guidera, 'USADA's Methods Seem Un-American'. *Savannah Morning News*, June 13, 2004. http://www.savannahnow.com/stories/061204/2233896.shtml
61 See ASADA from note 58 above.
62 McLaren, 'CAS Doping Jurisprudence', 11; Myler, 'How Much is Enough?', 11.
63 In particular, the work conducted by Houlihan, *Dying to* Win, on anti-doping policy implementation would be a useful starting point.
64 Yesalis *et al*. 'Incidence of Anabolic Steroid Use', 73.
65 C. Yesalis and M. Bahrke, 'Where There is a Will to Gain an Edge, Athletes Find a Way'. *The New York Times*, March 7, 2004, Section 8, 1.
66 Mazanov, 'Measuring Athlete Attitudes Towards Drugs in Sport'.
67 See commentary on WADA Code Article 2.1.1 earlier in this essay.
68 National Anti-Doping Organizations such as ASADA, USADA, Drug Free Sport NZ and UK Sport.
69 See Houlihan, *Dying to* Win, 179–80.
70 Since the time of writing there have been some changes made to the WADA Code, which were due to come into force on January 1, 2009. Some provisions referred to in this article will have changed slightly, and the relevance of some comments may vary accordingly.

References

Amos, A. 'Inadvertent Doping and the WADA Code: Can Athletes with a Cold Breathe Easy?' *Bond Law Review* 19, no. 2 (2007): 1.

'Arbitration CAS 95/142. *C v Fédération Internationale de Natation Amateur (FINA)*, award of April 22, 1996'. In *Recueil des sentences du TAS, Digest of CAS Awards II 1986–1998*, edited by Matthieu Reeb, 215–24. Berne: Staempfli Editions SA Berne, 1998.

Arbitration CAS 95/142. L v Fédération Internationale de Natation Amateur (FINA), 1995. In *Recueil des sentences du TAS, Digest of CAS Awards II 1986–1998*, edited by Matthieu Reeb, 225. Berne: Staempfli Editions SA Berne, 1998.

Arbitration CAS 94/129. USA Shooting & Q *v* International Shooting Union (UIT), award May 23, 1995. In *Recueil des sentences du TAS, Digest of CAS Awards II 1986–1998*, edited by Matthieu Reeb, 187–204. Berne: Staempfli Editions SA Berne, 1998.

Baxter v International Olympic Committee (IOC). 'Arbitration CAS 2002/A/376, award of October 15, 2002'. In *Recueil des sentences du TAS Digest of CAS awards III: 2001–2003*, edited by M. Reeb, 303. The Hague: Kluwer Law International, 2004.

Beloff, M. 'Drugs, Law and Versapaks'. In *Drugs and Doping in Sport: Socio-Legal Perspectives*, edited by J. O'Leary, 39–56. London: Cavendish, 2001.

Blair, F. 'Procedural Fairness in Doping Disputes'. *UNSW Law Journal* 22, no. 3 (1999): 885–93.

Briginshaw v Briginshaw. CLR 60 (1938): 336.

Buti, A. and S. Fridman. 'The Intersection of Law and Policy: Drug Testing in Sport'. *Australian Journal of Public Administration* 53, no. 4 (1994): 459–505.

Buti, A., and S. Fridman. 'Drug Testing in Sport: Legal Challenges and Issues'. *University of Queensland Law Journal* 20, no. 2 (1999): 153–85.

Buti, A., and S. Fridman. *Drugs, Sport and the Law*. Mudgeeraba: Scribbler's Publishing, 2001.

Ferstle, J. 'Evolution and Politics of Drug Testing'. In *Doping in Elite Sport: The Politics of Drugs in the Olympic Movement*, edited by W. Wilson and E. Derse, 363–413. Champaign, IL: Human Kinetics, 2001.

Fitzgerald, M. 'The Court of Arbitration for Sport; Dealing with Doping and Due Process during the Olympics'. *Sports Law Journal* 7 (2000): 213–35.

Foschi, J.K. 'A Constant Battle: The Evolving Challenges in the International Fight against Doping in Sport'. *Duke Journal of Comparative and International Law* 16 (2006): 457.

Mr Mark French v Australian Sports Commission and Cycling Australia. CAS 2004/A/651. Appeal Partial Award pronounced by the Court of Arbitration for Sport Oceania Registry, July 11, 2005.

Gasser v Stinson and Holt. Unreported, High Court of Justice Chancery Division, J. Scott, June 15, 1988. Cited in T. Kavanagh, 'The Doping Cases and the Deed for the International Court of Arbitration for Sport (CAS)'. *UNSW Law Journal* 22, no. 3 (2001): 721–45.

Grayson, E. 'Drugs, Sport and the Olympics'. *New Law Journal* 142 (1992): 1171.

He Kaw Teh v The Queen. (1985) 157 CLR 523.

Hatch, H. 'On Your Marks, Get Set, Stop! Drug Testing Appeals in the IAAF'. *Loyola and Los Angeles International and Comparative Law Journal* 16 (1994): 537–656.

Houlihan, B. *Dying to Win: Doping in Sport and the Development of Anti-Doping Policy.* Strasbourg: Council of Europe Publishing, 1999.

Kavanagh, T. 'The Doping Cases and the Need for the International Court of Arbitration for Sport (CAS)'. *UNSW Law Journal* 22, no. 3 (1999): 721–45.

Mazanov, J. 'Measuring Athlete Attitudes Towards Drugs in Sport'. In *Proceedings for the ACSPRI Social Science Methodology Conference 2006*, edited by J. Hanson and F. Quirk. Australia: ACSPRI, 2006.

Mbaye, K. 'Report of the Working Group on the Legal and Political Aspects of Doping.' Paper presented at the World Conference on Doping in Sport, Lausanne, February 2–4, 1999.

McLaren, R. 'Exceptional Circumstances: Is it Strict?' *International Sports Law Review* 2 (2005): 32–7.

McLaren, R. 'CAS Doping Jurisprudence; What Can we Learn?' *International Sports Law Review* 1 (2006): 4–22.

Melethil, S. 'Making the WADA Prohibited List: Show Me the Data'. *Saint Louis University Law Journal* 50 (2005): 75.

Modahl v The British Athletic Federation Ltd. Unreported, UK Court of Appeal, July 28, 1997.

Myler, C. 'How Much is Enough? Using Circumstantial Evidence to Prosecute Olympic-sport Athletes for Anti-doping Rule Violations'. *NYSBA Entertainment and Sports Law Journal* 16 (2005): 8–12.

National Wheelchair Basketball v International Paralympic Committee. CAS 95/122. In *Recueil des sentences du TAS, Digest of CAS Awards II 1986–1998*, edited by M. Reeb. The Hague: Kluwer Law International, 1998.

Nordenfelt v Maxim Nordenfelt Guns and Ammunition Co Ltd [1894] AC 535.

Olympic Movement Anti-Doping Code (OMAC). In *Doping Rules of International Sporting Organizations*, edited by R. Siekman, J. Soek and A. Bellani, 599–624. The Hague: TMC Asser Instituut, 1999.

Opie, H. 'Legal Regimes for the Control of Performance-enhancing Drugs in Sport'. *Adelaide Law Review* 12 (1990): 332.

Oschutz, F. 'Harmonization of Anti-doping Code through Arbitration: The Case Law of the Court of Arbitration for Sport'. *Marquette Sports Law Review* 12 (2002): 675.

Oschutz, F. 'Doping Cases before the CAS and the World Anti-Doping Code'. In *The Court of Arbitration for Sport 1984–2004*, edited by I.S. Blackshaw, R.C.R. Siekmann and J. Soek, 246–65. The Hague: TMC Asser Press, 2006.

Pate and Hall v Australian Professional Cycling Council Incorporated. Unreported, Supreme Court of Victoria, No. 9215216, settled out of court March 1992.

Mariano Puerta v International Tennis Federation (ITF). Arbitral Award Pronounced by Court of Arbitration for Sport. CAS 2006/A/1025.

Raducan, Andreea v International Olympic Committee (IOC). 'Arbitration CAS ad hoc Division (O.G. Sydney) 2000/011, award of 28 September 2000'. In *Recueil des sentences du TAS, Digest of CAS Awards II 1998–2000*, edited by M. Reeb, 665. The Hague: Kluwer Law International, 2002.

Reeb, M. *Recueil des sentences du TAS Digest of CAS Awards II: 1998–2000.* The Hague: Kluwer Law International, 2002.

Reeb, M. *Recueil des sentences du TAS Digest of CAS awards III: 2001–2003.* The Hague: Kluwer Law International, 2004.

Reynolds v International Amateur Athletics Federation. US District Court, Sth District of Ohio, Eastern Division, 3 December 1992.

Rigozzi, A., G. Kaufman-Kohler, and G. Malinverni. 'Doping and the Fundamental Rights of Athletes: Comments in the Wake of the Adoption of the World Anti-Doping Code'. *International Sports Law Review* 3 (2003): 39.

Robertson v Australian Professional Cycling Council Incorporated. 'Unreported, Supreme Court of NSW Equity Division, Waddell CJ, September 10, 1992'. Reported in *Drugs, Sport and the Law*, edited by A. Buti and S. Fridman, 127. Mudgeeraba: Scribbler's Publishing, 2001.

Giorgia Squizzato and Fédération International de Natation Amateur (FINA), CAS 2005/A/830. Arbitral Award Pronounced by the Court of Arbitration for Sport.

Straubel, M. 'Doping Due Process: A Critique of the Doping Control Process in International Sport'. *Dickinson Law Review* 106, no. 3 (2002): 523–72.

United States Anti-Doping Agency. 'Former World Champion Collins Receives Eight-year Suspension for Participation in BALCO Drug Conspiracy.' News Release, December 2004.

V v Internationale de Natation Amateur (FINA). 'CAS 95/150'. In *Recueil des sentences du TAS, Digest of CAS Awards II 1998–2000*, edited by M. Reeb, 265. The Hague: Kluwer Law International, 2002.

Verroken, M. 'Drug Use and Abuse in Sport'. In *Drugs in Sport*, 4th ed., edited by D.R. Mottram, 29–63. New York: Routledge, 2005.

Vinnicombe v Australian Sports Drug Agency. Unreported decision, Federal Court of Australia, NSW District Registry, No G00065 of 1992.

Yesalis, C.E., M.S. Bahrke, A.N. Kopstein, and C.K. Barsukiewicz. 'Incidence of Anabolic Steroid Use: A Discussion of Methodological Issues'. In *Anabolic Steroids in Sport and Exercise*, 2nd ed., edited by C. Yesalis, 73–115. Champaign, IL: Human Kinetics, 2000.

Health psychology and drugs in sport

Frances H. Quirk

School of Arts and Social Sciences, James Cook University, Queensland, Australia

Health psychology, as a discipline in the social sciences, has the potential to make significant contributions to our understanding of the issue of performance enhancement in sport. This includes providing additional methods for deriving epidemiological and prevalence data, exploration of motives, decision-making and contributing contextual factors and the application of models of behaviour and methodologies that are aligned with health psychology. The application of theory is a major component of health psychology practice and occurs at the primary, secondary and tertiary level of intervention, which has parallels within performance enhancement in sport with prevention and detection. The use of different sampling methods and frames and aspects of health psychology clinical practice can broaden our understanding of the factors that contribute to identifying the elements of decision making and behaviour in performance enhancement in sport and have potential to contribute to the development of risk profiles and effective interventions.

When considering the contribution of health psychology to drugs in sport research we can immediately identify areas of current application and future potential. Some of these areas have been realised in practice, such as the principles of health education and health promotion in the conveyance of information about the risks to health of substance use in the context of sport. More specific contributions include assessment of mood, personality, coping style and attitudes as potential predictors of distress, response to injury, and compliance with anti-doping policy. Whilst there has been some publication of work in these areas, they are surprisingly few in number and the focus of psychological input is more on improving performance, coaching relationships and attitudes about drug use in sport than an in-depth exploration of motives, decision-making and contributing contextual factors. Few authors have transferred the knowledge base of health psychology to add to the methodological and theoretical approaches of this issue. As an example, there has been limited application of the models identified above in the specific arena of compliance with anti-doping policy. There are some areas which do seem to be intuitively appropriate, particularly health behaviours, coping strategies and substance use and also some clinical approaches which may be of relevance. These areas form the basis of the discussion of health psychology and drugs in sport.

How health psychology sees the world

Health psychology is a relatively recent development in the discipline of psychology, with its primary focus being the understanding of how the behaviour of the individual influences their health. For example, how aspects of personality may influence health (e.g. pessimism and heart disease[1]). Matarazzo's definition of health psychology tells us that health psychology is the 'aggregate of the specific education, scientific and professional contribution of the discipline of psychology to the promotion and maintenance of health, the promotion and treatment of illness, and related dysfunction'.[2]

An analysis of Ogden's view of health psychology suggests the sub-discipline has two primary functions, the first of which is the *development of theory*.[3] The broad aims of health psychology in this regard include:

- evaluating the role of behaviour in the aetiology of illness,
- predicting unhealthy behaviours,
- evaluating the interaction between psychology and physiology, and
- understanding the role of psychology in the experience of illness.

Ogden's approach to health psychology suggests the second primary function stems from the role of evaluating how psychology engages with the treatment of illness; that is, *putting theory into practice* by:

- promoting healthy behaviour through increased understanding of the role of behaviour in illness and targeting unhealthy behaviours,
- preventing illness by changing beliefs and behaviour,
- modifying stress,
- providing psychoeducation, and
- identifying behavioural intentions to promote recovery and facilitate behaviour change.

Using Matarazzo and Ogden's ideas, health psychology can be broadly characterized as a discipline seeking to further the understanding of attitudes, values, beliefs and motivations around decisions that have associated health risks, such as taking substances (like performance-enhancing drugs), and identifying the steps of the decision-making process leading to those behaviours. This is where the ideas of primary, secondary and tertiary prevention become important to health psychology.

Health psychology has a significant interest in primary prevention, or encouraging people to avoid behaviours we know carry health risk, such as the effort to help young people navigate adolescence without developing a smoking habit. Health psychology does this by looking at what biological, psychological, social and cultural factors contribute to an adolescent's decision to start smoking; there is ample scope for this effort to be repeated for drugs in sport. Health psychology is also interested in secondary prevention. Following the adolescent smoking example, this is where an adolescent has started smoking and health psychology tries to find ways to get them to change their behaviour by augmenting the decision process to stop. Finally, health psychology is interested in tertiary prevention, or how to help people cope with the illness they have. An example of this is when an adolescent who kept smoking develops, say, emphysema. Health psychology looks to helping them adapt their behaviour to live with the illness.

What health psychology has done

A literature search of terms that link sport and health psychology leads to a surprisingly low yield and can be summarized under the following headings: coping, personality, mood, stress and attitudes to drug use.[4] Often, linking terms are not actually addressing the issue of drug use but predictive factors relating to performance, recovery from injury, response to injury and coaching relationships. Many publications use adolescents or college athletes as their population sample which leads us to question how generalizable these findings would be to elite athletes competing at international competition standards.

Contextualizing drugs in sport for health psychology

Before applying the theory and methods of health psychology to the issue of drugs in sport, it is important to get a sense of the social context in which drugs in sport exists. For example, asking questions about how many athletes are using and the sorts of drugs they are using become important background information. Thus, the epidemiology of drugs in sport is an important part to developing health psychology's approach to this area.

Prevalence

The 2005 'out of competition' testing data collected and reported by the World Anti-Doping Agency (WADA) show that of 3,114 athletes tested, there were 61 adverse results (1.9%). From July 2004 to June 2005, the Australian Sport and Anti-Doping Agency (ASADA) reported that of 3,764 athletes, there were 16 registered offences (0.4%). The United States doping agency, (USADA), report a similar Figure (0.2%). Aggregate studies of prevalence rates over time suggest that 2% or below is a fairly stable estimate of the proportion of athletes tested who will return a reportable offence.[5]

Official testing reported by FIFA shows that the incidence rate within football (soccer) was an average 0.12% over 11 years, with prevalence of 0.42% in 2004 and 0.37% in 2005.[6] The same report goes on to admit that they actually have no idea of the true extent of performance-enhancing drug (PED) use in football. Outside official testing, projective techniques estimate that PED use among professional English footballers (soccer players) is around 6%.[7] This figure was derived using a projective technique asking how many professional footballers knew someone who used PEDs and working back to the estimate. While this may be inflated,[8] it is certainly higher than official figures.

The further away from official estimates one gets, the higher the supposed incidence rates. The anecdotal evidence of a much wider prevalence rate exists, with American baseball and American football, weight lifting and cycling often cited as examples of sports where use is more common than abstinence. According to Morgan anecdotal estimates range from 5%–95%.[9] While these figures are unreliable, they do suggest that the plausible range of prevalence estimates extends from FIFA's 0.12% all the way to 95%. Looking at this with a critical eye, it confirms Dvorak *et al.*'s admission that no one really has any idea of the true prevalence of drugs in sport. The British Medical Association (BMA) goes one step further, declaring that 'the true extent of doping in sport is unknown'.[10] This lack of firm evidence for prevalence rates forms a significant gap in knowledge for health psychology, social science and science more broadly.

Social Factors: Who is performance enhancement a problem for?

The national and international agencies, whose manifestos establish their position against performance enhancement in sport, communicate very clear messages about the compromising effects of performance enhancement in sport. There is some question as to whether the general public, sports fans, media, medical profession, athletes and sports personnel adhere to the same viewpoint. This is a largely unexplored area, although studies in Europe suggest that athletes themselves would be more inclined to introduce harsher penalties for illegal performance enhancement.[11]

Some researchers[12] take the view that PED use is more closely aligned to criminal behaviour and that athletes (and sports personnel) make conscious decisions, having weighed up the costs and benefits, to maximize their best interests. This 'criminalizing' of performance enhancement may lead to changes in perceptions amongst the general public and sports fans.

Hughes and Coakley suggested that this is 'positive deviance' and a result of over-conformity to the norms and values embodied in sport.[13] These authors argued that the espoused 'sport ethic' of commitment, sacrifice for the 'game', seeking distinction, taking risks and challenging limits lead athletes to be vulnerable to the facilitative ability of performance enhancement to meet this 'ethic'. This suggestion has been endorsed in a series of interviews with 50 steroid users, aged between 15 and 40 years, in which one of the rationalizations for abusing steroids was given as 'a code of commitment to sport'.[14] Black takes this evidence one step further to argue that the ban on performance enhancement achieves the opposite of its intended outcome and that most deaths and injuries occurring during the ban would not have occurred in the absence of it.[15] This suggests performance enhancement is the lesser problem compared to sports participation and over-enthusiastic adherence to the 'sport ethic'.

In their discussion paper of the social construction of drug debates, Dingelstad and colleagues suggest that the current stance in sport reflects the dominance of sports administrators as the major interest group in the performance enhancement in sport debate.[16] It is in the interest of the International Olympic Committees (IOCs) and national sports administrative agencies to promote sport as an 'arena of fair competition' and to be seen to be actively pursuing the image of sport as fair, and drug testing is a way to protect this image. The reality of professional sport in contemporary society is that it is big business driven by the mass media and corporations – the espousing of 'fair play' is an image left over from the days of amateur competition which has less and less to do with the reality of professional sport.[17] As Dingelstad *et al.* argue, 'drug use has increased as sport has become dominated by business interests and (in the Olympics) a matter of government prestige'.[18]

Carstairs examined the media and public response to doping scandals and noted that it is more difficult to access the responses of sports fans and the general public than those more immediately involved, such as, sports journalists, administrators and athletes themselves.[19] This is an area that is particularly ripe for exploration utilizing social science research methodology (e.g. surveys, qualitative interviews and focus groups).

The drugs in sport context

In summary, the context for drugs in sport research appears to be both real and imagined. The reality is that drugs in sport do exist, and that some athletes do use to achieve some advantage as a result; just how many is at issue. The problem of estimating actual prevalence rates means that any number is plausible, from the negligible to the anxiety invoking. The reality is that the sports industry (championed by the IOC) cares about drugs in sport. The vested interest means that this may be more of an issue for the sports industry than the general public. What is central here is that contextualizing drugs in sport for health psychology has already led to two questions that need to be on the research agenda for a social science on drugs in sport: prevalence and public opinion.

Theories and models of health behaviour

Health psychology has a lot of ways of conceptualizing health behaviour when examining drugs in sport. The three overarching concepts from health psychology are examined here. The first relates to the social cognitive theories and models as a way to explain PED use. The second looks at drug use as a response to occupational stress experienced by elite or professional athletes. The third and final overarching concept used is addiction.

Social cognition

As a discipline, health psychology has contributed a great deal to our knowledge of health behaviour and behaviour change. These contributions vary from the development of theoretical models of behaviour to the development of interventions that aim to improve attendance at health screening programmes or engagement in positive or protective health behaviours. These models are dominated by the social cognition approach to understanding decision making (e.g. the intention to do more exercise) and subsequent behaviour (actually going to the gym). In essence these models look at how decisions people make to change or maintain health behaviours based on a cost-benefit analysis (e.g. threat to health *versus* performance outcome) arise from their perception of information (e.g. perceived vulnerability and severity of risk) and interpretation of their social environment (e.g. attitudes and what other people think). The most prominent of these theories of behavioural change and intention to change include the Health Belief Model (HBM), the Theory of Planned Behaviour (TPB) and the Health Action Process Approach (HAPA).[20]

Social cognition models define a range of factors that contribute to the probability of changing behaviour (or behavioural intention) and have been moderately successful in predicting the choices of individuals in terms of health behaviours.[21] Models of health behaviour and behavioural intention may have the most applied utility in contributing to an understanding of choices and contextual factors around compliance and non-compliance with doping policy. Donovan, Egger, Kapernick and Mendoza incorporated behavioural science frameworks in their sports drug compliance model and identified six major inputs to an athlete's intentions surrounding performance enhancement.[22] Of the six, five represented elements of various social cognition behaviour change models: threat appraisal, benefit appraisal, reference group influences, personal morality and legitimacy. The final element related to personality factors.

Where social cognition struggles

One of the issues with framing performance enhancement in sport within a social cognition typology or, more specifically, as a health behaviour amenable to intervention, is an underlying assumption that PED use is perceived as a negative action with consequent health risks. This is conceptualized as a threat appraisal. When the health risk is apparent, the social cognition models assume the threat to health as motivating towards abstention. This leads to a rather important question of whether athletes engaging in performance enhancement view taking PEDs as negative. As part of answering this question, the social cognition approach requires some insight into whether athletes understand and actually consider the potential health consequences before they decide to use. This is essentially asking whether the health consequences of using PEDs influence athletes' decision to use PEDs. Tracking this one step further, a more fundamental question for health psychology is whether athletes even consider performance enhancement as a form of health behaviour.[23]

There is some evidence that a 'win at all costs' mentality overrides the basic tenets of a health behaviour model that assumes people are motivated to protect their health from PEDs. Jacobs and Samuels[24] report a study where a Chicago doctor asked 198 Olympic-level athletes whether they would take a drug that was undetectable if the drug meant a certain win. Of the 198 asked, only two responded negatively. In response to an additional question asking the same athletes if they would consider taking the same drug for five years if it meant certain wins for five years but then certain death caused by the side effects, more than half of the sample indicated that they would. Traditional health belief and health behaviour models have trouble explaining this apparent acceptance of health risk and mortality, unless we view them from a different perspective. If the outcome is viewed, from the athletes' perspective, as success in competition rather than engagement in health behaviour, then performance enhancement becomes a natural feature of the model and the decision sequence; engaging in performance enhancement is driven by necessity to meet the functional goal of success in competition.

Using HAPA to describe athlete PED use

The HAPA is a reconciliation of prominent social cognitive models of health behaviour, such as the HBM and TPB. The HAPA identifies:

- an initial motivation phase, where the person develops an intention to act based on the relative influence of three predictors of change (perceived self efficacy, outcome expectancies and risk perception);
- a phase where plans to act are formulated (intentions);
- trying to act; and,
- effort and persistence towards maintaining or disengaging the behaviour.

Perceived self-efficacy is a predictor of success for each stage of the model and efficacy beliefs determine appraisal of personal resources in stressful encounters and contribute to the forming of behavioural intentions.

We now track an athlete's theoretical progression through the HAPA to illustrate how it explains PED use in athletes. Initially, the outcome expectancy is related to an understanding of training, nutrition and supplementation within legal parameters leading to success. Risk perception may relate to the probability of injury or being in competition against another athlete with a better personal best. Perceived self-efficacy might be related to prior performance, confidence in the coach and training programme. The intention and planning stages may focus on training, rehabilitation, nutrition support, engaging a good coach/trainer, time management, stress management with a goal of successful competition and a win. However, if with all of these in place and commitment and engagement being evident the outcome is something other than what the athlete perceives as 'success', then the athlete's personal model about getting to the desired outcome needs to be reviewed. Perhaps perceived self-efficacy is supplemented by enhanced self-efficacy through some form of performance enhancement method. Outcome expectancies are increased in relation to use of a 'guaranteed' method, risk perception (threat appraisal) now includes the risk of being caught and exposed as a 'cheat' leading to intention and planning to accessing the performance enhancer and maintaining secrecy. The athlete (or associated sports personnel) becomes a learning organism and makes good use of readily available resources to ensure the desired outcome.

When viewed in this way, performance enhancement, whether by drugs, supplementation or other methods, is a natural consequence of either experience or knowledge of contextual factors (i.e. other athletes are presumed to be enhancing their performance) and is perceived as an adaptive response rather than a maladaptive one in meeting the goal of winning. Donovan *et al.* refer to this as a 'reversal' of HBM concepts.[25] Constructs such as decisional balance, ambivalence, self-efficacy, situational temptation and perceived reward for effort are all factors that derive from the application of HAPA to the drugs in sport context that might affect transitions between contemplation, intention and action phases of behaviour change. These may also be factors worth exploring in the context of determining athletes behaviour or developing interventions.

Stress and strain

The notion of effort-reward imbalance is a conceptualization of work stress[26] that may be relevant to athletes who view their role in performance sport as a 'job' or career. This is particularly true for elite athletes and sports persons who may well commit the majority of their teenage and young adult lives to sports training and participation.[27]

Whilst there has been some focus on coping with acute stress in a sporting context, for example, how Rugby League players respond to intense or stressful events during a match,[28] there has been little exploration of the impact of chronic stress for athletes in the pressured and success-focussed environment of elite competition. The other main research on stress in sport has been on the relationship between stress and injury, and some evidence that 'life events' can influence the risk of injury. Whilst this may be buffered by social support, there is also evidence of readiness to take risks on the part of injured athletes and this may reflect sensation-seeking traits (lack of caution, adventurous spirit and drive for excitement/tension). However, there is no evidence of an 'injury-prone' athlete personality profile[29] which might increase athletes' vulnerability to PED use for recovery or rehabilitation.

Davids, Smith and Martin[30] present an applied psychological framework for coping with performance uncertainty in sport and work systems and identified that a theme of personal control serves as a link between the ideas promoted in the stress literature and organizational psychology. The focus was on learned resourcefulness and the promotion of tacit knowledge in the individual. Linking back to the previous section on health behaviours we might speculate that a decision to use performance-enhancing drugs or methods is an example of learned resourcefulness, where increasing the certainty of performance is a significant motivator. This line of reasoning is consistent with other viewpoints that performance enhancement in the sporting context is inevitable.[31] This represents a possible line of research to demonstrate that anti-doping is perhaps a less effective way of managing the role of drugs in sport and that other avenues need to be explored.

Addiction

The basic premise of this section examines whether illegal and PED use reflect an underlying addictive or dependent personality. There is certainly scope for considering PED use alongside the use of other addictive drugs (e.g. nicotine, amphetamines or heroin). Laure, Thouvenin and Lecerf's[32] study on the attitudes of General Practitioners in France showed the majority considered PED use as a form of drug addiction. The argument is presented in two ways. The first is through co-morbidity, where PED use exists alongside the abuse of other addictive substances. The second is the possibility that PED use is an artefact of an addiction to sport.

Co-morbidity

A number of studies have examined the co-occurrence of performance-enhancing drug use and recreational drug use, with mixed results. Lorente, Peretti-Watel and Grelot investigated the concurrent use of cannabis in French sport university students and found that male students were prone to already have used cannabis to enhance non-sporting and sporting performance.[33] This relationship was bi-directional and dependent on both level of competition and the type of sport. Peters *et al.* investigated the beliefs and norms associated with ephedra use and perceived addiction among university athletes in the Southwest of the United States of America using a qualitative design. Of those participants who self identified as users, the majority perceived that addiction was established by routine behaviour and was perpetuated by the negative consequences of stopping use. These consequences were related to the perceived reasons for starting use and differed between male and female students. Male students reported difficulty with stopping due to the consequent decrease in athletic performance, sickness and weight gain. Female students were more concerned about the impact on their appearance, i.e. weight gain.[34]

A second French study suggested that participating in performance enhancement and drug use whilst being an athlete was a risk factor for developing dependence at the end of a sporting career.[35] The study explored level of sporting activity and drug use and dependence amongst outpatient attendees at health centres and support groups for alcohol and heroine use. Of the 1,111 questionnaires completed, 10% of respondents had participated in sport at national or international level competition. Within this group, 36% reported intravenous drug use and 16% that they had already used doping substances; however only 28% stated that they experienced dependence during the period of high level competition. This was relative to 15% who described dependence before this period and a much greater proportion afterwards (56%). The authors concluded that a high level sports training could not be viewed as protective in terms of drug addictive behaviours and that competitive athletes may be particularly at risk for drug use and addiction at the end of their careers. It is important to note that the population under study in this research is biased in terms of being recruited as outpatients with dependency or addiction problems. Acknowledging this, the prevalence of drug and substance use amongst the athlete group does suggest that athletes may develop dependency as a result of their chosen careers rather than having a dependent or addictive profile which leads to drug use in competition. The authors suggest that more studies are needed to evaluate individual vulnerability factors, the effects of overtraining and to determine the periods when youths who are participating in sport are most likely to abuse drugs.

Addicted to sport

It is also possible that sports participation itself might be considered a kind of 'drug' and that the compulsive and obsessive commitment and training, associated with positive feedback from success and the positive endorsements of others may be a motivation to choose other drug pathways as a way of maintaining that success and positive reinforcement.[36] Reviews of the presenting problems of the athlete clients of clinical and counselling psychologists suggest that substance-related disorders were one of the primary areas of psychopathology covered in individual therapy.[37] If the elite athlete could be considered in this way, then it may be possible to conceive of this group as possessing a pathology of performance enhancement of which PEDs form one part.[38] That is, such athletes may be statistically abnormal in the way they perceive the world and process information (with attendant implications for models of social cognition) that lead to disordered thinking about PED use.

Other Factors

Unlike the discussion of theories and models above, this section focuses on variables that health psychology has learned are useful in exploring a range of behaviours. Three are explored. The first looks to the influence of body image. The second is whether a personality typology might be developed to explain variations in PED vulnerability and use. The third looks to the influence of significant others on PED use behaviour.

Body image

A central question relates to what rewards individuals participating in performance enhancement in sport derive, apart from the perception of increasing competitive edge. Some studies have suggested that there may be gendered attributions that contribute to the perception of rewards, especially as regards body image.

Research by Ricciardelli, McCabe and Banfield examined the role of sport to understand adolescent males' views about their body.[39] In the first study semi-structured interviews were conducted with 40 adolescent boys aged between 15 and 17 years. Thematic analysis of the narratives generated in interviews showed that sport provided these adolescent boys with a context for discussing their body image, and attributes which males liked about their body were synonymous with those associated with being successful at sport. In addition, sport was used as an opportunity for competing with other males both through the playing of sport and by using sport performance to make favourable social comparisons about their body size. Additional gender influence was noted in a second study by Ricciardelli, McCabe and Ridge where feedback from mothers and female friends were viewed as having a positive impact on boys' body image and feed-back from fathers and male friends was viewed as more important in influencing body change methods.[40] The media was also viewed as contributing to boys' body satisfaction but it was seen to encourage greater exercise to alter body size and shape.

Genetic and physical limitations in body size and shape may act as promoters of willingness to explore alternative methods of acquiring the desired body, muscle bulk or performance to achieve positive feedback. Monaghan's qualitative exploration of motives for illicit drug use amongst bodybuilders suggested that the three main justifications for steroid use were; self-fulfilment (steroid use was rationalized as a legitimate means to an end), condemnation of condemners (negative judgments from others were rejected) and denial of injury (bodybuilders claimed that steroids do not seriously harm the user's health or threaten society more generally).[41] These subjective meanings serve to provide a framework of justification for engaging in illicit substance use. This identifies a potential avenue of exploration for health psychologists in determining the subjective meanings for athletes in engaging in performance-enhancing drug use.

Whilst in Monaghan's sample the subjective justifications provide the rationale for steroid use, there is evidence that steroid use does have negative health consequences of significance. Abuse of anabolic steroids has been associated with psychiatric and medical effects and there appears to be a dose response relationship between increased doses of steroid and the severity of psychiatric symptomatology, although the true extent of the contribution of androgenic-anabolic steroid abuse to violence and behavioural disorders is unknown.[42] Psychological factors may also be considered as potentially causal for anabolic steroid use as some research has identified disturbance in body image (body dysmorphia) as a factor in initiating use of steroids.[43] Other predictors include the use of other drugs (multiple drug use), engaging in strength training, being male and alcohol use.[44]

A disturbing thought is that performance enhancement in sport could be related to performance enhancement in image. Some researchers refer to the general group of performance-enhancing substances as 'performance and image enhancing drugs'. There are also reports that younger athletes are increasingly experimenting with both illicit substances and nutritional supplements to improve performance *and* appearance.[45] This suggests that there may be some overlap between the psychology of performance enhancement in sport and image enhancement (such as cosmetic surgery) that may be worth exploring.

Personality

The development of a 'doping typology' is an attractive option in the early identification of individuals at risk of doping behaviour and enhancing prevention of drug use in sport. However, a doping 'personality profile' has been elusive. Burnett and Kleiman[46] used a personality inventory and mood profile to assess psychological characteristics in three groups of adolescents:

- athletes who reported steroid use,
- athletes who did not use steroids, and
- non-athletes.

There were some personality differences between athletes and non-athletes but no significant ones between athletes who were steroid users and those who did not use steroids. There were physical difference betweens steroid users and non-users in terms of muscular density, gynaecomastia and acne, but mood differences, such as depression and anger, were only detectable between steroid users on a use cycle versus steroid users not on a use cycle.

Porcerelli and Sandler looked more specifically at narcissism and empathy in weightlifters and bodybuilders and compared those who did use anabolic steroids with those who did not.[47] Steroid users had significantly higher scores on dimensions of pathological narcissism and significantly lower empathy scores; the authors note that it is unclear whether narcissistic personality traits contribute to the use of anabolic steroids or are a consequence of steroid use. These data suggest that personality may be a less important predictor of doping behaviour. However, more longitudinal studies are required to increase our understanding of the psychological issues involved in both adolescent and adult steroid use before any firm claim can be made.

Raglin[48] revisited the Mental Health Model of sports performance, which claims that there is a correlation between psychopathology and performance; as an athlete's mental health declines so does their performance. The model also suggests the converse is also true, that as an athlete's mental health improves so does their performance. Studies have identified that a high proportion (70–85%) of successful and unsuccessful athletes can be predicted from measures of personality structure and mood. Longitudinal data has shown that as training load increases mood decreases and that this may lead to an increase in 'staleness syndrome' for athletes who are undergoing intensive training for an upcoming competition. This observed relationship may also contribute to the possibility of performance-enhancement practices as a form of 'self-medication' to avoid or alleviate the depressed mood associated with performance decline. As demonstrated in Petrie and Diehl's reviews of problems athletes present when consulting clinical and counselling psychologists, anxiety, stress and depressive disorders were amongst the primary areas of psychopathology.[49]

Seligman identified that the traits of optimism and pessimism in elite athletes may be related to risk of non-compliance and that this predictive pathway was mediated by self-esteem.[50] Athletes with a more optimistic personality style tended to attribute success to their own personal efforts and failure to external, specific and temporary factors, such as poor refereeing, illness or the weather. As the optimistic athlete operates within an understanding that their success is their own and failure is not, he/she tends to have robust levels of self-esteem. Athletes with a more pessimistic personality style tended to attribute failure to more personal and general factors, such as lack of skill and lack of motivation. This tendency to attribute failure to 'self' leads to reduced self-esteem. Seligman hypothesized that athletes who attribute poor performance or failure to internal, stable and generalized personal factors would be more likely to engage in performance enhancement to 'overcome' these perceived disadvantages.

Significant others

Athletes are situated within an 'organizational' framework that includes WADA, national level agencies, sports' training institutions, trainers, coaches, peers, family and friends. Each of these agencies convey attitudes, beliefs, principles and values which may have more or less bearing on the athlete's own attitudes and behaviour in relation to performance enhancement.

To adequately address the issue of performance enhancement in sport (or any other issue in the competitive sporting arena) a multi-dimensional, multi-layer, complex systems approach lends itself to determining the interaction of both implicit and explicit agents (organizational, group, and individual) and the biological, psychological and social pressures that lead to illegal performance enhancement.

One of the possible contextual factors exerting social pressure for athletes in their decision making around drug use is the attitude of coaches and trainers to performance enhancement. An evaluation of professional coaches' attitudes in France[51] indicated that, of the 260 coaches who responded:

- 10% considered an athlete could use doping with no health hazard with the help of a physician,
- 30% indicated that athletes who decline doping had no hope of succeeding,
- 6% had used doping drugs in the previous 12 months, and
- 13.5% of coaches reported that athletes told them they had been prompted to use doping drugs in the previous 12 months.

The coaches' attitudes to current anti-doping prevention were negative, with approximately 80% considering that current methods ineffective and that they (the coaches) were poorly trained to prevent doping.

Streigel *et al.*[52] looked at athlete's views in Germany and the research indicated that the active participation of athletes themselves would be the most effective mechanism for further improvement and success of anti-doping measures. Of the 101 athletes interviewed, 98% agreed that action should be taken against doping in sport, although improved detection methods and increased information provision of health risks were supported more than increasing the severity of punishments. Participants also indicated that they would be willing to be tested more frequently, despite the privacy infringements involved. Of course, there is some issue with the reliability and validity of such results given the sensitivity of the issues and the potential willingness of athletes to say what they think people want to hear.

Supplement use

Where the focus has largely been on PEDs, there is likely to be another avenue for exploring the use of performance-enhancing substances more generally, namely performance-enhancing supplements. These supplements are used by the general population due to a perception they enhance general health or have some protective effect against illness (e.g. taking Vitamin C, garlic, horseradish or Echinacea supplements to protect against colds or influenza). There are also a range of supplements that are perceived to have performance-enhancing effects of interest to athletes, such as protein, creatine or ginseng.

Supplement use may be a useful proxy for PED use. In fact, a significant number of athletes use supplements for their perceived performance-enhancing effects. At the elite level, more than half of UK athletes had used such supplements (60%).[53] While most supplement users did so to avoid illness (the reason given by 63% of supplement users), there was clearly a performance-enhancing element to the use, with maintaining strength (38%) and enhancing endurance (20%) the second and third most common reasons. Metzl, Levine and Gershel suggest that as many as 28% of collegiate athletes admit taking a popular performance enhancing supplement, creatine.[54] Reasons given for taking creatine were enhanced performance (74%) and improved appearance (61%), and the most common reason for not taking creatine was safety (45% of non-users).

In fact, there is epidemiological evidence from university-level athletes[55] that those using supplements are more than four times more likely to report using PEDs. This result is limited by the self-report nature of the study and the fact its results may be unreflective of what elite athletes do. However, it does suggest there is a link between supplement use and PED use which might be exploited by researchers. A significant advantage for studying drugs in sport through supplements is that athletes may be more forthcoming about their supplement use. This would allow for the development of a model of performance-enhancement *substance* use, rather than PED use.[56]

Specific techniques and methods

Health psychology, as an applied discipline, has a number of research methods and techniques that may have utility both in describing what factors contribute to the choice to use performance enhancement and the development of interventions to deter or detect this non-compliance with the current anti-doping rules. The approach of health psychology is different to that taken by other psychology disciplines and the techniques and applied frameworks reported here draw from health promotion, health behaviour research, epidemiology and clinical practice.

Sampling frames

The utility of research relevant to the performance enhancement in sport debate lies in the sampling frame. One important element that needs to be included is representation from the major agencies interested in drugs in sport (e.g. government, policy makers, clubs, officials, player's unions, athletes, fans and members of the public disinterested in sport). This allows for the development of a detailed and rich understanding of the contributing factors and issues from a variety of different perspectives. Taking such an approach necessitates the application of the cutting edge tools available to describe both the elements and the structure of such complex systems, possibly including structural equation modelling or micro-simulations of behaviour. Such detailed analysis from multiple perspectives throws light on the complexity of the issue and identifies common threads or themes that can be further explored employing quantitative and qualitative research methods.

Survey/self-report questionnaires

Survey methodology can be more or less sophisticated depending on the resources available and the research question of interest. Surveys, often presented in the form of a paper 'questionnaire' with varying response options or a telephone assisted interview, are a method of inferring a population opinion, attitude or set of beliefs by randomly sampling individuals within the population. This is where the precise definition of the sampling frame outline above becomes important. The methods for sampling participants vary in relation to access and demands of the project as does the way the survey is conducted. Examples of modes of surveying populations include, computer-assisted personal interview (CAPI), computer-assisted telephone interview (CATI) and self-administration (e.g. via mail or over the internet).

Whilst the form of questionnaire is most often used to generate inferences or estimates about the population, questionnaires also have other applications. A well designed and appropriately validated questionnaire can also be employed to generate hypotheses, to get a feel for how people respond to certain issues (e.g. 'should performance enhancement in sport be banned?') or to see if there are any underlying factors that appear to be influencing how people respond to a set of questions (e.g. the level of affiliation to professional sport determining the strength of opinion about banning performance enhancement). Questionnaires can also be employed to test causal models (e.g. specific personality factors are related to non-compliance with anti-doping regulations), confirm ideas about differences between specific groups (e.g. weightlifters are more frequent users of anabolic steroids than ballet dancers) or to evaluate an intervention (e.g. education programme about the health risks of performance enhancement).

These methods have utility in researching the question of motivations, attitudes, beliefs and behaviour in relation to performance enhancement in sport, exemplified by the articles cited in this review. Quantitative data has been the most commonly presented, although there is an opportunity to broaden the methodological approach by increasing the use of qualitative methods.

Clinical approaches: motivational interviewing

Health behaviour research suggests that interventions addressing motivation can enhance the likelihood of behavioural change and the translation of intention into action.[57] Before behaviours change individuals need to be motivated to do so. Motivational Interviewing (MI) is a therapeutic technique employed to facilitate behaviour change when individuals are engaging in negative health behaviours (e.g. substance abuse).[58] Aspects of MI may have utility in exploring factors that contribute to PED use and the attitudes and motivations of athletes and sports personnel to be compliant or non-complaint with anti-doping policy.

MI has been employed in clinical populations to effect change in substance use, compliance with medication regimes and eating behaviour. The main aim of MI is to facilitate behaviour change by enhancing intrinsic motivation and bringing an individual to awareness of ambivalence around behaviour change, encouraging the individual to develop insight into the costs and benefits of maintaining or changing a particular behaviour. The identification of ambivalence allows individuals to examine their motivations and needs for engaging in behaviours that they or others would like them to change.

One method for explicitly identifying ambivalence is a Decisional Balance Sheet (DBS): individuals are asked to consider the costs and benefits of maintaining the behaviour and the costs and benefits of ceasing the behaviour. The benefits of maintaining the behaviour and the costs of ceasing it contribute the most to ambivalence about change. MI identifies three factors that are contingent to behaviour change, the *willingness* to change, the *ability* to change and the *readiness* to change. The DBS process can contribute to determining, for an individual, whether they are *willing*, *able* and *ready* (WAR) to change their behaviour and also what factors need to change for them to meet these motivational requirements. These three factors are consistent with components of health-related behaviour models (e.g. HAPA), where *willingness* and *ability* are akin to elements of the predictive phase of behavioural change (e.g. outcome expectancies, perceived self-efficacy, risk perception) and *readiness* to change is equated with intention and planning (e.g. the Transtheoretical Model).[59] The action phase of behavioural change in the HAPA model is strongly associated with perceived self efficacy (*ability*) and this element is a focus of the MI therapeutic process. MI aims to increase self worth, self-esteem and confidence through expressing empathy, giving praise and clarifying ambivalence. This process supports individuals making changes in their behaviour by enhancing motivation and self-efficacy. Moreover, it explicitly identifies the factors contributing to the maintenance of the behaviour and prevention of behaviour change.

MI has clear theoretical links to social cognition models of health behaviour change, and especially the HAPA. The HAPA identifies factors that contribute to behavioural intentions and the implementation of intentions in action and strongly supports the notion of self efficacy as predictive of behavioural intention and subsequent action. The HAPA and MI can also be linked at the applied level in terms of experimental methodology and design, where a focus on understanding and enhancing the factors that contribute to self-efficacy (and identifying factors that undermine self-efficacy) would be translated into outcome (i.e. compliance with anti-doping policy).

It is proposed that aspects of MI and specifically the DBS process have utility in highlighting issues and factors that contribute to decisions to use PEDs in sport, and also the issues and factors that contribute to decisions to abstain. The focus would be on participants' perceptions of issues and factors that contribute to *willingness*, *ability* and *readiness* (WAR) to change performance enhancement behaviour or to maintain compliance with, for example, anti-doping regulations. There might be application in asking how athletes would respond to alternative forms of regulation to drugs in sport to get a sense of what would be most effective in relation to their behaviour. Applying the MI techniques within each of the major interest groups in professional sport, including sports fans and the general public, would generate a substantive body of information relating to perceptions of attitudes, beliefs and motivations around performance enhancement in sport, and may help clarify discrepancies in assumptions about performance enhancement within and between these groups.

What health psychology needs to know

The use of performance-enhancing drugs or methods has become more widespread as athletes and sports personnel continue to look for ways to gain a competitive edge, or at least keep up with the competition. The drugs and methods of choice change over time as more 'evidence', perceived or actual, becomes available to support or disconfirm their efficacy. The use of multiple substances or methods is common, although the impact on performance and health of multiple combinations is not always known.[60] The motives for engaging in performance enhancement have not been fully explored and as Donovan *et al.* note in their review article, the limited research falling within a social science framework has focussed more on athletes' attitudes about performance enhancement than their motivations.[61] Of the six major elements identified by these authors identified as likely influences on an athlete's attitudes and intentions towards performance enhancement, the first four (personality factors, threat appraisal, benefit appraisal and reference group influences) are already clearly identified in contemporary models of health behaviour as contributing to decision making around choices relating to health and behaviour that influence or impacts on health. However, as has already been identified, these models may operate 'in reverse' when considering the issue of performance enhancement. What is crucial, though, is the absence of any empirical data supporting these theoretical contentions.

At the general level, this review suggests a number of possibilities both in terms of factors potentially contributing to non-compliance with anti-doping regulations and methods and approaches to further explore and address this issue. It is clear, however, that these factors are at the personal, group, structural and organizational level within professional sport and that the approach and appropriate methodologies must be selected to address this multi-factorial, multi-dimensional problem.

A research agenda for health psychology

1. Using sampling frames that take into account a range of groups with an interest in sport to explore and increase knowledge of the subjective contributions of agency and the meaning of performance in sport; particularly so for the general public and athletes themselves.
2. Establishing a clear epidemiology of drugs in sport, making use of broadly defined sampling frames. As part of this, work on the relationship between PED and nutritional supplement use is needed.
3. Employing techniques used in clinical health psychology practice, such as Motivational Interviewing, to provide additional insights and practical methods to test whether theories

and models of health behaviour are an appropriate way of conceptualizing athlete responses to drugs in sport.

4. Studies on elite athlete populations to assess the predictive nature of variables identified in the theories and models of health behaviour, and also to confirm or disconfirm results from amateur or collegiate sporting contexts.
5. Performance enhancement in sport needs to be addressed as a 'systems' issue. Athletes are one component of the system and dependent on the other components. Analytical methods which accommodate complex structural systems, such as structural equation modelling or micro-simulations, may be usefully employed to explore system structure and the relative contribution of various components to athlete (and other interest group) decision making about drugs in sport.

Notes

1 Sarafino, *Health Psychology*.
2 Matarazzo, 'Behavioural Health and Behavioural Medicine', 815.
3 Ogden, *Health Psychology*.
4 LeUnes and Burger, 'Bibliography on the Profile of Mood States in Sport and Exercise'; Moss, Panzale and Tarter, 'Personality, Mood and Psychiatric Symptoms among Anabolic Steroid Users'; Nilsson *et al.*, 'Attitudes and behaviours with regards to androgenic anabolic steroids'; Peters *et al.*, 'Beliefs and Social Norms about Ephedra Onset and Perceived Addiction among College Male and Female Athletes'.
5 Mottram, *Drugs in Sport*.
6 Dvorak *et al.*, 'FIFA's Approach to Doping in Football'.
7 Waddington *et al.*, 'Drug Use in English Professional Football'.
8 Yesalis, Kopstein and Bahrke, 'Difficulties in Estimating the Prevalence of Drug Use among Athletes'.
9 Morgan, 'Fair is Fair, or is it?'
10 BMA, *Drugs in Sport*, 87.
11 Streigel, Vollkommer and Dickhuth, 'Combating Drug Use in Competitive Sports'.
12 Strelan and Boeckmann, 'A New Model for Understanding Performance-enhancing Drug Use by Elite Athletes', and Strelan and Boeckmann, 'Why Drug Testing in Elite Sport Does not Work'.
13 Hughes and Coakley, 'Positive Deviance among Athletes'.
14 Fuller and LaFountain, 'Performance-enhancing Drugs in Sport'.
15 Black, 'Does the Ban on Drugs in Sport Improve Societal Welfare?'
16 Dingelstad *et al.*, 'The Social Construction of Drug Debates'.
17 Rosner and Shropshire, *The Business of Sports*.
18 Dingelstad *et al.*, 'The Social Construction of Drug Debates', 1833.
19 Carstairs, 'The Wide World of Doping'.
20 The Health Belief Model from Becker and Rosenstock, 'Compliance with Medical Advice'; the Theory of Planned Behaviour from Ajzen and Madden, 'Prediction of Goal-directed Behaviour'; the Health Action Process approach from Schwarzer, 'Social-cognitive Factors in Changing Health-related Behaviours'.
21 Albarracin *et al.*, 'Theories of Reasoned Action and Planned Behaviour as Models of Condom Use'; Armitage and Conner, 'Efficacy of the Theory of Planned Behaviour'; Hagger, Chatziserantic and Biddle, 'A Meta-analytic Review of the Theories of Reasoned Action and Planned Behaviour in Physical Activity'; Hausenblas, Carron and Mack, 'Application of the Theories of Reasoned Action and Planned Behaviour to Exercise Behaviour'; Weinstein, 'Testing Four Competing Theories of Health-protective Behaviour'.
22 Donovan *et al.*, 'A Conceptual Framework for Achieving Performance Enhancing Drug Compliance in Sport'.
23 O'Donnell, Mazanov and Huybers, 'Towards a Choice Model of Athletes' Decision to use Performance Enhancing Substances or Methods'.
24 Jacobs and Samuels, 'The Drug Testing Project in International Sports'.
25 Donovan *et al.*, 'A Conceptual Framework for Achieving Performance Enhancing Drug Compliance in Sport'.
26 Siegrist, 'Adverse Health Effects of High Effort/Low-reward Conditions'.
27 Brissonneau, 'Deviant Careers: The Case of Cycling'.
28 Anshel, 'Qualitative Validation of a Model for Coping with Acute Stress in Sport'.

[29] Bianco, 'Social Support and Recovery from Sport Injury'; Junge, 'The Influence of Psychological Factors on Sports Injuries'.
[30] Davids, Smith and Martin, 'Controlling System Uncertainty in Sport and Work'.
[31] Savulescu, Foddy and Clayton, 'Why We Should Allow Performance Enhancing Drugs in Sport'; Haugen, 'The Performance Enhancing Drug Game'.
[32] Laure, Thouvenin and Lecerf, 'Attitudes of Coaches towards Doping'.
[33] Lorente, Peretti-Watel and Grelot, 'Cannabis Use to Enhance Sportive and Non-sportive Performances among French Sport Students'.
[34] Peters *et al.*, 'Beliefs and Social Norms'.
[35] Lowenstein *et al.*, 'Physical and Sports Activities in the History of Patients Treated for Addictions'.
[36] Dunning and Waddington, 'Sport as a Drug and Drugs in Sport'.
[37] Petrie and Diehl, 'Sport Psychology in the Profession of Psychology'; Petrie, Diehl and Watkins, 'Sport Psychology: An Emerging Domain in the Counselling Psychology Profession?'
[38] Mazanov, O'Donnell and Battley, 'Psychology and Drugs in Sport'.
[39] Ricciardelli, McCabe and Banfield, 'Body Image and Body Change Methods in Adolescent Boys'.
[40] Ricciardelli, McCabe and Ridge, 'The Construction of the Adolescent Male Body through Sport'.
[41] Monaghan, 'Vocabularies of Motive for Illicit Steroid Use among Bodybuilders'.
[42] Chyka, 'Health risks of Selected Performance-enhancing Drugs'; Pope and Katz, 'Psychiatric and Medical Effects of Anabolic-androgenic Steroid Use'; Porcerelli and Sandler, 'Narcissism and Empathy in Steroid Users'.
[43] Wroblewska, 'Androgenic-anabolic Steroids and Body Dysmorphia in Young Men'.
[44] DuRant, Escobedo and Heath, 'Anabolic-steroid Use, Strength Training, and Multiple Drug Use'.
[45] Calfee and Fadale, 'Popular Ergogenic Drugs and Supplements in Young Athletes'; Congeni and Miller, 'Supplements and Drugs Used to Enhance Athletic Performance'.
[46] Burnett and Kleiman, 'Psychological Characteristics of Adolescent Steroid Users'.
[47] Porcerelli and Sandler, 'Anabolic-androgenic Steroid Abuse and Psychopathology'.
[48] Raglin, 'Psychological Factors in Sport Performance'.
[49] Seligman, *Learned optimism.*
[50] Petrie and Diehl, 'Sport Psychology in the Profession of Psychology'.
[51] Laure, Thouvenin and Lecerf, 'Attitudes of Coaches towards Doping'.
[52] Striegel, Vollkommer and Dickhuth, 'Combating Drug Use in Competitive Sports'.
[53] UK Sport, *2005 Drug Free Survey.*
[54] Metzl, Levine and Gershel, 'Creatine Use among Young Athletes'.
[55] Papadopoulos *et al.*, 'Doping Use among Tertiary Education Students'.
[56] Mazanov *et al.*, 'Towards an Empirical Model of Performance Enhancing Supplement Use'.
[57] Jackson *et al.*, 'Beyond Intention: Do Specific Plans Increase Health Behaviours in Patients in Primary Care?'; Rothman and Salovey, 'Shaping Perceptions to Motivate Healthy Behaviour: The Role of Message Framing'.
[58] Miller and Rollnick, *Motivational Interviewing.*
[59] Prochaska and DiClemente, 'Transtheoretical Therapy'.
[60] Boyce, 'Use and Effectiveness of Performance-Enhancing Substances'.
[61] Donovan *et al.*, 'A Conceptual Framework'.

References

Ajzen, I., and T. Madden. 'Prediction of Goal-directed Behaviour: Attitudes, Intentions and Perceived Behavioural Control'. *Journal of Experimental Social Psychology* 22 (1986): 453–74.

Albarracin, D., B. Johnson, M. Fishbein, and P. Muellerleile. 'Theories of Reasoned Action and Planned Behaviour as Models of Condom Use: A Meta-analysis'. *Psychological Bulletin* 127 (2001): 142–61.

Anshel, M. 'Qualitative Validation of a Model for Coping with Acute Stress in Sport'. *Journal of Sport Behaviour* 24 (2001): 223–46.

Armitage, C., and M. Conner. 'Efficacy of the Theory of Planned Behaviour: A Meta-analytic Review'. *British Journal of Social Psychology* 40 (2001): 471–99.

Becker, M., and I. Rosenstock. 'Compliance with Medical Advice'. In *Health Care and Human Behaviour*, edited by A. Steptoe and A. Mathews, 175–208. London: Academic Press, 1984.

Bianco, T. 'Social Support and Recovery from Sport Injury: Elite Skiers Share their Experiences'. *Research Quarterly for Exercise and Sport* 72 (2001): 376–88.

Black, T. 'Does the Ban on Drugs in Sport Improve Societal Welfare?' *International Review for the Sociology of Sport* 31 (1996): 367–84.

BMA. *Drugs in Sport: The Pressure to Perform*. UK: BMJ Publishing Group, 2002.
Boyce, E. 'Use and Effectiveness of Performance-Enhancing Substances'. *Journal of Pharmacy Practice* 16 (2003): 22–36.
Brissonneau, C. 'Deviant Careers: The Case of Cycling'. Paper presented at the WADA Conference on Ethics and Social Science Research in Anti-doping, Larnaca, Cyprus, April 13–14, 2006.
Burnett, K., and M. Kleiman. 'Psychological Characteristics of Adolescent Steroid Users'. *Adolescence* 29 (1994): 81–9.
Calfee, R., and P. Fadale. 'Popular Ergogenic Drugs and Supplements in Young Athletes'. *Pediatrics* 117 (2006): 577–89.
Carstairs, C. 'The Wide World of Doping: Drug Scandals, Natural Bodies and the Business of Sports Entertainment'. *Addiction Research and Theory* 11 (2003): 262–81.
Chyka, P. 'Health Risks of Selected Performance-Enhancing Drugs'. *Journal of Pharmacy Practice* 16 (2003): 37–44.
Congeni, J., and S. Miller. 'Supplements and Drugs Used to Enhance Athletic Performance'. *Paediatric Clinicians of North America* 49 (2002): 435–61.
Davids, K., L. Smith, and R. Martin. 'Controlling System Uncertainty in Sport and Work'. *Applied Ergonomics* 22 (1991): 312–5.
Dingelstad, D., R. Gosden, B. Martin, and N. Vakas. 'The Social Construction of Drug Debates'. *Social Science and Medicine* 43 (1996): 1829–38.
Donovan, R., G. Egger, V. Kapernick, and J. Mendoza. 'A Conceptual Framework for Achieving Performance Enhancing Drug Compliance in Sport'. *Sports Medicine* 32 (2002): 269–84.
Dunning, E., and I. Waddington. 'Sport as a Drug and Drugs in Sport: Some Exploratory Comments'. *International Review for the Sociology of Sport* 38 (2003): 351–68.
DuRant, R., L. Escobedo, and G. Heath. 'Anabolic-steroid Use, Strength Training, and Multiple Drug Use among Adolescents in the United States'. *Pediatrics* 96 (1995): 23–8.
Dvorak, J., T. Graf-Baumann, M. D'Hooghe, D. Kirkendall, H. Taennler, and M. Saugy. 'FIFA's Approach to Doping in Football'. *British Journal of Sports Medicine* 40 (2006): i3–i12.
Fuller, J., and M. LaFountain. 'Performance-enhancing Drugs in Sport: A Different Form of Drug Abuse'. *Adolescence* 22 (1987): 969–76.
Hagger, M., N. Chatzisarantic, and S. Biddle. 'A Meta-analytic Review of the Theories of Reasoned Action and Planned Behaviour in Physical Activity: Predictive Validity and the Contribution of Additional Variables'. *Journal of Sport and Exercise Psychology* 24 (2002): 3–32.
Haugen, K. 'The Performance Enhancing Drug Game'. *Journal of Sports Economics* 5 (2004): 67–86.
Hausenblas, H., A. Carron, and D. Mack. 'Application of the Theories of Reasoned Action and Planned Behaviour to Exercise Behaviour: A Meta-analysis'. *Journal of Sport and Exercise Psychology* 19 (1997): 36–51.
Hughes, R., and J. Coakley. 'Positive Deviance among Athletes: The Implications of Overconformity to the Sports Ethic'. In *Contemporary Issues in Sociology of Sport*, edited by A. Yiannakis and M. Melnick, 361–74. Champaign, IL: Human Kinetics, 2001.
Jackson, C., R. Lawton, P. Knapp, D. Raynor, M. Conner, C. Lowe, and S. Closs. 'Beyond Intention: Do Specific Plans Increase Health Behaviours in Patients in Primary Care? A Study of Fruit and Vegetable Consumption'. *Social Science and Medicine* 60 (2005): 2383–391.
Jacobs, J., and B. Samuels. 'The Drug Testing Project in International Sports: Dilemmas in an Expanding Regulatory Regime'. *Hastings International and Comparative Law Review* 18 (1995): 557–89.
Junge, A. 'The Influence of Psychological Factors on Sports Injuries. Review of the Literature'. *American Journal of Sports Medicine* 28 (2000): S10–S15.
Laure, P., F. Thouvenin, and T. Lecerf. 'Attitudes of Coaches Towards Doping'. *Journal of Sports Medicine and Physical Fitness* 41 (2001): 132–6.
LeUnes, A., and J. Burger. 'Bibliography on the Profile of Mood States in Sport and Exercise, 1971–1995'. *Journal of Sport Behaviour* 21 (1998): 53–70.
Lorente, F.O., P. Peretti-Watel, and L. Grelot. 'Cannabis Use to Enhance Sportive and Non-sportive Performances among French Sport Students'. *Addictive Behaviour* 30 (2005): 1382–91.
Lowenstein, W., P. Arvers, L. Gourarier, A. Porche, J. Cohen, F. Nordmann, B. Prevot, C. Carrier, and M. Sanchez. 'Physical and Sports Activities in the History of Patients Treated for Addictions'. *Annals de Medicine Interne* (Paris) 151, Suppl. A (2005): A18–A26.
Matarazzo, J. 'Behavioural Health and Behavioural Medicine: Frontiers for a New Health Psychology'. *American Psychologist* 35 (1980): 807–17.

Mazanov, J., T. O'Donnell, and A. Battley. 'Psychology and Drugs in Sport: The Annoyed, the Inspired and the Road Ahead'. *The Sporting Mind* 5 (2006): 3–8.

Mazanov, J., A. Petroczi, J. Bingham, and A. Holloway. 'Towards an Empirical Model of Performance Enhancing Supplement Use: A Pilot Study among High Performance UK Athletes'. *Journal of Science and Medicine in Sport* 11 (2008): 185–90.

Metzl, J., S. Levine, and J. Gershel. 'Creatine Use Among Young Athletes'. *Pediatrics* 108 (2001): 421–5.

Miller, W., and S. Rollnick. *Motivational Interviewing: Preparing People for Change*, 2nd ed. New York: Guildford Press, 2002.

Monaghan, L. 'Vocabularies of Motive for Illicit Steroid Use among Bodybuilders'. *Social Science and Medicine* 55 (2002): 695–708.

Morgan, W. 'Fair is Fair, or is it?: A Moral Consideration of the Doping Wars in American Sport'. *Sport in Society* 9 (2006): 177–98.

Moss, H., G. Panzale, and R. Tarter. 'Personality, Mood and Psychiatric Symptoms among Anabolic Steroid Users'. *The American Journal of Addictions* 1 (1992): 315–24.

Mottram, D.R. *Drugs in Sport*, 4th ed. New York: Routledge, 2005.

Nilsson, S., F. Spak, B. Marklund, A. Baigi, and P. Allebeck. 'Attitudes and Behaviours with Regards to Androgenic Anabolic Steroids among Male Adolescents in a County of Sweden'. *Substance Use and Misuse* 40 (2005): 1–12.

O'Donnell, T., J. Mazanov, and T. Huybers. 'Towards a Choice Model of Athletes' Decision to Use Performance Enhancing Substances or Methods: Factors and Covariates'. Paper presented at the ACSPRI Social Science Methodology Conference 2006. Australia, ACPSRI.

Ogden, J. *Health Psychology: A Textbook*. Milton Keynes: Open University Press, 2004.

Papadopoulos, F., I. Skalkidis, J. Parkkari, E. Petridou and 'Sports Injuries' European Union Group. 'Doping Use among Tertiary Education Students in Six Developed Countries'. *European Journal of Epidemiology* 21 (2006): 307–13.

Peters, R., L. Adams, J. Barnes, L. Hines, D. Jones, K. Krebs, and S. Kelder. 'Beliefs and Social Norms about Ephedra Onset and Perceived Addiction among College Male and Female Athletes'. *Substance Use and Misuse* 40 (2005): 125–35.

Petrie, T., and N. Diehl. 'Sport Psychology in the Profession of Psychology'. *Professional Psychology: Research and Practice* 26 (1995): 288–91.

Petrie, T., N. Diehl, and C. Watkins. 'Sport Psychology: An Emerging Domain in the Counselling Psychology Profession?' *The Counselling Psychologist* 23 (1995): 535–45.

Pope, H., and D. Katz. 'Psychiatric and Medical Effects of Anabolic-androgenic Steroid Use. A Controlled Study of 160 Athletes'. *Archives of General Psychiatry* 51 (1994): 375–82.

Porcerelli, J., and B. Sandler. 'Narcissism and Empathy in Steroid Users'. *American Journal of Psychiatry* 152 (1995): 1672–4.

Porcerelli, J., and B. Sandler. 'Anabolic-androgenic Steroid Abuse and Psychopathology'. *Psychiatric Clinicians of North America* 21 (1998): 829–33.

Prochaska, J., and C. DiClemente. 'Transtheoretical Therapy: Toward a More Integrative Model of Change'. *Psychotherapy: Theory Research and Practice* 19 (1982): 276–88.

Raglin, J. 'Psychological Factors in Sport Performance: The Mental Health Model Revisited'. *Sports Medicine* 31 (2001): 875–90.

Ricciardelli, L., M. McCabe, and S. Banfield. 'Body Image and Body Change Methods in Adolescent Boys: Role of Parents, Friends and the Media'. *Journal of Psychosomatic Research* 49 (2000): 189–97.

Ricciardelli, L., M. McCabe, and D. Ridge. 'The Construction of the Adolescent Male Body through Sport'. *Journal of Health Psychology* 11 (2006): 577–87.

Rosner, S., and K. Shropshire. *The Business of Sports*. Sudbury, MA: Jones and Bartlett Publishers, 2004.

Rothman, A., and P. Salovey. 'Shaping Perceptions to Motivate Healthy Behaviour: The Role of Message Framing'. *Psychological Bulletin* 121 (1997): 3–19.

Sarafino, E. *Health Psychology: Biopsychosocial Interactions*, 5th ed. New York: John Wiley, 2006.

Savulescu, J., B. Foddy, and M. Clayton. 'Why We Should Allow Performance Enhancing Drugs in Sport'. *British Journal of Sports Medicine* 38 (2004): 666–70.

Schwarzer, R. 'Social-cognitive Factors in Changing Health-related Behaviours'. In *Current Directions in Health Psychology*, edited by G. Miller and E. Chen, 157–63. Upper Saddle River, NJ: Prentice Hall, 2005.

Seligman, M. *Learned Optimism*. New York: Pocket Books, 1991.

Siegrist, J. 'Adverse Health Effects of High Effort/Low-reward Conditions'. *Journal of Occupational Health Psychology* 1 (1996): 27–41.

Streigel, H., G. Vollkommer, and H. Dickhuth. 'Combating Drug Use in Competitive Sports. An Analysis from the Athletes' Perspective'. *Journal of Sports Medicine and Physical Fitness* 42 (2002): 354–9.

Strelan, P., and R. Boeckmann. 'A New Model for Understanding Performance-enhancing Drug Use by Elite Athletes'. *Journal of Applied Sport Psychology* 15 (2003): 176–83.

Strelan, P., and R. Boeckmann. 'Why Drug Testing in Elite Sport Does Not Work: Perceptual Deterrence Theory and the Role of Personal Moral Beliefs'. *Journal of Applied Social Psychology* 36 (2006): 2909–34.

UKSport. *2005 Drug Free Survey*. London: UKSport, 2006.

Waddington, I., D. Malcolm, M. Roderick, and R. Naik. 'Drug Use in English Professional Football'. *British Journal of Sports Medicine* 39 (2005): e18.

Weinstein, N. 'Testing Four Competing Theories of Health-protective Behaviour'. *Health Psychology* 12 (1993): 324–33.

Wroblewska, A. 'Androgenic-anabolic Steroids and Body Dysmorphia in Young Men'. *Journal of Psychosomatic Research* 42 (1997): 225–34.

Yesalis, C., A. Kopstein, and M. Bahrke. 'Difficulties in Estimating the Prevalence of Drug Use among Athletes'. In *Doping in Elite Sport: The Politics of Drugs in the Olympic Movement*, edited by W. Wilson and E. Derse, 43–62. Champaign, IL: Human Kinetics, 2001.

Equipping athletes to make informed decisions about performance-enhancing drug use: a constructivist perspective from educational psychology

James M. Hanson

School of Business, UNSW@ADFA, Canberra, Australia

This essay introduces some prominent constructivist theories of learning and shows how they can be applied to the design of anti-doping education programmes. It briefly outlines the ATLAS and ATHENA programmes, which have had some success in the USA, and explores the potential for educational research to make further contributions to the development of successful anti-doping education programmes. Recommended directions for future research into the education of athletes about performance-enhancing drug use include evaluation of existing educational interventions, testing just how much athletes know about drugs in sport, and whether educational programmes need evolve with the maturing athlete to impact their drug use behaviour.

Education has been given a central role by national anti-doping organisations (NADOs) as a method of deterring athletes from using performance-enhancing drugs (PEDs). However, over the last 30 years, research in human cognition and learning has shown that designing *effective* education programmes is a far greater challenge than had long been assumed.[1] Traditional teaching, which treated education as information transmission, learning as memorizing, teachers as subject-matter experts and learners as passive audience members, has increasingly given way to newer approaches which view education as knowledge construction, learning as guided investigation, teachers as model investigators and students as co-investigators. Although these new, constructivist approaches can be found in schools and some universities, state-of-the-art knowledge about human thinking and learning has rarely been incorporated into the design and delivery of anti-doping education programmes. Educational research has the potential to change this situation for the better.

Education is, strictly speaking, not a single discipline. Educational research, like health research or management research, draws upon multiple academic disciplines – philosophy, sociology, history, anthropology, economics and psychology, to name but a few. It also draws upon all other disciplines in the form of educational content. While philosophers, historians and sociologists have tended to address questions about the ‘what’ and ‘why’ of education, psychologists and, increasingly, anthropologists have tended to focus on the ‘how’ of education – the processes or practices of human learning. Educational psychology investigates human learning with a view to developing interventions that may enhance learning or shape it in particular ways.

How an educational perspective sees the world

In democratic societies, the role of education is not only to inform learners of prevailing, hopefully research-based, views about the nature of the physical and social world, but also to equip those learners to make informed decisions and to subject beliefs – their own and those espoused by others – to critical evaluation. It is this concern for enhancing personal autonomy, rather than merely securing uncritical compliance, that many constructivists regard as distinguishing liberal education from authoritarian propaganda. These 'constructivist values' in education are summarized by Lebow as: 'collaboration, personal autonomy, generativity, reflectivity, active engagement, personal relevance and pluralism'.[2]

When presented with the opportunity to use PEDs, athletes make a decision. However, they may or may not engage in the search for information, critical evaluation of that information and the reflective weighing up of pros and cons that we can loosely label 'rational' decision making. A constructivist educational agenda would seek to equip athletes with the skills and attitudes required to actively consider the options and potential consequences of their decisions and to evaluate the validity of the information and advice that they are being offered. It would also seek to investigate the prevailing beliefs among athletes about the effects and the desirability of using PEDs and to challenge those beliefs on both scientific and ethical grounds so that they can be articulated and subjected to examination, debate and reflection. This does not guarantee that athletes will come to view PEDs in a uniformly negative light or that all athletes will choose not to use them under any circumstances, but, if successful, it ought to ensure that athletes do not simply drift unreflectively and uncritically into the practice of using PEDs.

Recognizing that, in democratic societies, athletes have autonomy to make their own decisions about PED use, Donovan, Egger, Kapernick and Mendoza place athletes' attitudes or intentions regarding PED use at the centre of their sport drug control model.[3] In their model, athletes' attitudes are influenced by six factors: threat appraisal, benefit appraisal, personal morality, perceived legitimacy, reference group opinion and personality/self-esteem. Attitudes, in turn, are posited to influence drug use behaviours, subject to the affordability and availability of substances.

Athletes' beliefs or perceptions are treated as crucial, in this model, because it is their subjective *beliefs* about threats and benefits, about what is to be regarded as the right thing to do, about the legitimacy of drug-related organizations and about the opinions of key reference groups that shape their attitudes.

Educational research can, perhaps, make its most useful contribution to this issue, by: (1) designing and evaluating interventions that challenge and improve the validity of athletes' existing beliefs, and (2) designing and evaluating interventions that equip athletes with the skills and critical attitudes to evaluate, for themselves, the validity of claims made about the consequences of using PEDs.

This essay outlines the main theoretical principles of the constructivist view of human learning and some empirical research findings that clarify what constructivist approaches to education look like, in practice. Furthermore, these theoretical principles and research findings are applied to the ATLAS and ATHENA programmes – two drug and health-related education programmes which have been shown to achieve some positive impacts on athletes in American high-school sport teams.[4] Finally, it will explore more general conclusions about the potential role of anti-doping education programmes.

What the educational perspective has done

ATLAS and ATHENA: case studies of drugs in sport education

ATLAS was a programme developed to educate adolescent male athletes about the use of anabolic steroids.[5] ATHENA was a programme developed, using the same principles, to educate adolescent female athletes about substance use and eating disorders.[6] The programmes are designed around interactive peer-based education in the context of sports teams. Members of the teams nominated to become squad leaders were trained and took responsibility for running the largely-scripted programme, facilitated by coaches or trainers, as needed. The sessions involved discussions of issues relevant to substance use and eating disorders, creating health promotion media and role plays. Factual material was provided to participants via booklets. Empirical data from the studies shows that this programme reduced participants' reported actual use, and intentions to use, performance-enhancing substances, such as steroids and amphetamines, and other substances, such as alcohol, tobacco and marijuana, up to three years after the intervention.[7]

Developing learners' understanding of concepts (beliefs): constructivist views of learning

The development of learners' conceptual understanding has been a long-standing educational objective. However, it is an objective that has not often proved easy to achieve. Although traditional didactic approaches to instruction (i.e. via chalk, talk and textbook) have been successful in developing the ability of learners to memorize and recall factual statements and to perform routine procedures, these achievements, in themselves, do not necessarily indicate conceptual understanding.

Traditional teaching

Dissatisfaction with traditional teaching, via knowledge transmission, is based on empirical evidence that, although didactic teaching is *intended* to facilitate learners' general understanding of concepts, learners frequently fail to achieve such understanding.[8] Memorization, recitation and symbolic manipulation of definitions and statements that express the meanings of concepts in general terms are not synonymous with understanding those concepts. Learners taught didactically often show little proficiency in applying the concepts to make decisions or in recognizing situations where the concepts could be used for interpretation and explanation. This is the age-old problem of inert knowledge – knowledge that can be recited but not readily recalled in relevant situations or applied to problems.[9]

Indeed, studies have shown that learners who have pre-existing misconceptions about a topic can also learn a scientifically-accepted alternative without ever challenging their pre-existing beliefs. In a sense, they have two separate knowledge structures for different purposes. They use the scientifically-sanctioned concepts to answer test or exam questions, but naively continue to use their earlier misconceptions to make judgements in day-to-day life.[10]

In light of these findings, it would not be surprising for an athlete to memorize and recount, in good faith, any number of statements about the ineffectiveness or immorality of using a banned substance and yet still use that substance when the opportunity arises for want of applying those 'known' facts at the time of decision. Although the athlete may have memorized the facts, their meaning may not have been made personal, their practical implications not truly internalized.

Constructivist teaching

Constructivists in educational psychology are concerned with *meaning*: that is, with the development of a learner's personal understanding of conceptual knowledge. Their central assumption, based in Piagetian psychology, is that one's own understanding of conceptual knowledge is personally-constructed via reflection upon one's own experiences, so the task of educators is to engage with learners' existing conceptions, provide learners with appropriate experiences and the means for interpreting them so as to restructure those existing conceptions or construct new ones. Constructivism posits that learning conceptual knowledge more inductively, by engaging with well-chosen, relevant problems, can ground or 'anchor' a person's understanding of those concepts in meaningful experience and facilitate the recall and application of knowledge in relevant situations.

Constructing an understanding of a concept requires two forms of engagement: direct engagement with the material or social systems to which the concept is relevant, and engagement with other learners to discuss, compare and possibly share their developing understandings of the concept and its applicability to those systems. In constructivist learning environments, learners must be both intellectually active and interactive.

Direct engagement with the material or social systems to which a concept is relevant is often achieved by the use of cases, problems, scenarios, simulations and experiments. As the learner's conceptual understanding develops, these may progress from simpler examples, which are designed to clearly illustrate the properties of the concept, toward more complex applications in which the concept may be used to make inferences and judgements about a realistic system or situation.[11] However, not all constructivist learning environments are organized this way. Some, such as Problem-Based Learning in medical education, use cases and problems of realistic complexity from the beginning.

Constructivist education programmes targeting athletes' use, or potential use, of PEDs might usefully be framed around realistic scenarios that begin by placing the learner in the position of decision-maker. Scenarios might involve a hypothetical colleague or teammate who has confided in the athlete that he or she is considering using a banned substance or, perhaps, a trainer approaching the athlete in a gym offering advice about where to acquire a banned substance and how to mask its use. The purpose of the scenarios would be to highlight the personal relevance of the information to be learned and to place its application squarely within a decision-making context. Of course, designing scenarios that are credible and relevant to the learner requires an understanding of how, when, where and by whom young athletes are likely to be presented with opportunities to use PEDs.

Two theories of learning

Two theories of cognitive development have been most influential in shaping constructivist pedagogy: Jean Piaget's personal constructivist theory of development via assimilation and accommodation,[12] and Lev Vygotsky's social constructivist theory of development via internalization and externalization of mediational tools, such as language, mathematical symbols, scientific diagrams and so on.[13] Their practical consequences for constructivist pedagogy are frequently in agreement and where they are not in agreement, they can often (although not always) be viewed as complementary rather than competing.

Piaget's personal constructivism is built on the processes of assimilation and accommodation – terms borrowed from biology. Human learners are viewed as organisms engaged with their environment. Learners build cognitive structures or 'schemes' through their interaction with the world and their actions on objects in the world. Moderately-novel experiences are related to familiar ones by assimilation; that is, they are interpreted according to existing cognitive schemes. However, genuinely novel experiences require accommodation – the construction of a new scheme into which the novel experience can be assimilated. The period of adjustment is characterized by cognitive conflict and disequilibrium and eventually, through resolution of the tension between assimilation and accommodation the learner achieves equilibration. The cognitive conflict and eventual equilibration in Piaget's personal constructivism can be regarded as analogous with the tension between empirical results and theory in a scientific discipline. New empirical findings may be satisfactorily explained by existing theories (i.e. assimilation) or they may require accommodation in the form of theoretical change. Indeed, Piaget's picture of the individual learner is that of the scientist experimenting in the world and either interpreting his observations via assimilation with existing schemes or, if necessary, accommodating unexpected findings by constructing new schemes.

Piaget also assigned an important role to social interaction. When learners compare their understandings of a given concept or a system to which the concept may apply, they will most likely find discrepancies between schemes that they have each constructed individually. This can provide a further source of conflict or disequilibrium, termed socio-cognitive conflict, which may lead each individual into further internal struggle between assimilation and accommodation. Whereas pure assimilation would involve retaining one's pre-existing scheme, interpreting the peer's belief in terms of one's own and pure accommodation would mean simply adopting the peer's belief as a new scheme, active engagement in socio-cognitive conflict may lead the learner to construct a new scheme that can reconcile the pre-existing views. Piaget regarded learners as most likely to engage in socio-cognitive conflict during interaction between peers of approximately equal status. Interactions involving unequal status too often lead to pure assimilation on the part of the higher status participant and pure accommodation on the part of the lower status participant.

The potential lesson for drug education programmes would be to design structured opportunities for debate and discussion among peers of equal status in which athletes are challenged safely to voice their existing beliefs so that those beliefs can be tested (e.g. ATLAS and ATHENA). Learning is as much about discarding or modifying old beliefs as it is about constructing new ones.

Vygotsky's social constructivism posits that a learner constructs higher psychological structures via internalization and externalization of symbolic tools, such as language, mathematical symbol systems, maps, scientific diagrams and the like.[14] Of these, internalization has received more attention among Vygotskians in the western world. Learners can internalize the use of semiotic tools (symbols) which are initially encountered in the external environment where they serve interpersonal functions of communication or sense-making. Some accounts depict internalization as little more than knowledge transmission but Vygotsky's own account emphasizes that internalization is not synonymous with copying.[15] Internalization is more akin to reconstruction in that it draws on the individual's experiences and prior knowledge – an account that is not so far from Piaget's.

Where Piaget and Vygotsky do differ is in the role that language and dialogue play in cognitive development. Piaget regarded thought and language as being related but quite distinct, whereas Vygotsky, following Dewey, regarded language as the principal tool of higher-order thinking. Thus, for Piaget, language is a means by which people may compare the results of their thinking while, for Vygotsky, language use is central to thinking in two ways: (1) higher-order thought operates via inner speech and is, therefore, disciplined by language, and (2) externalization in audible speech for others requires that thoughts be more precisely analysed and concepts carefully elaborated. From the Vygotskian perspective, our use of semiotic tools is not merely able to reflect knowledge schemes, but to construct them.

The role of externalization, in the Vygotskian approach, has received less attention, but it may be even more important to the construction of understanding than internalization. Externalization is the creation, using symbolic tools, of an external representation of a concept and through creating the external representation the concept may be restructured. Expressing a holistic thought in a sequential string of meaningful words and sentences is both an analytical and a creative act. For Vygotskians, knowledge construction and representation, or explanation, are activities that go hand in hand.

It is this link between knowledge construction and knowledge representation, or explanation, that places collaborative learning at the heart of Vygotskian social constructivist pedagogy. Where Piaget saw explanation as a means of comparing the products of individual thought, Vygotskian social constructivists see it as central to the process of thought, itself. It is in the struggle to depict, explain and elaborate the intimation of an idea that the idea is structured and clarified and knowledge is constructed – not only the external representation but also the internal cognitive structure. In constructing a conceptual representation with or for others, learners reconstruct the concepts for themselves.

One aspect of the ATLAS programme resonates clearly with these ideas. Athletes work in small groups to design a public-information campaign. Friendly competition among the groups encourages creativity in this design task so that learners are not simply repeating the messages that they were taught. Instead, they struggle to articulate the learned principles in new ways, requiring them to engage in deeper cognitive processing.

Engaging learners in solving authentic problems: constructivist programme design

In education programmes based on constructivist or social constructivist principles, direct transmission of knowledge from instructors to learners is regarded as problematic. Therefore, the main task of educators is the design of the learning environment. Simply confronting groups of learners with a problem is not sufficient to facilitate constructivist learning. Effective constructivist learning environments require learners to be both intellectually active and interactive. The active intellectual engagement of learners in constructing knowledge requires sustained effort which is more likely when the learners' intrinsic motivation or interest has been harnessed. This has ramifications for the design and selection of tasks or problems that comprise the experiential aspect of the constructivist programme. Likewise, the constructive interaction of learners requires that particular patterns of learner discourse and dialogue be modelled and encouraged. Not all forms of conversation are likely to result in the construction of valid conceptual knowledge. Principles for shaping learner activity and interactivity are discussed below. Although they are treated separately, it is important to note that both are necessary.

Constructivist instructional design principles for fostering active intellectual engagement among learners are outlined by Dunlap and Grabinger, and by Savery and Duffy, who list eight design principles for constructivist learning environments:[16]

1. all learning activities should be anchored to a larger task or problem rather than presented as stand-alone activities,
2. the learner should be supported in developing ownership of the larger task or problem possibly by soliciting problems from learners themselves or by designing and selecting problems that are likely to appeal to learners as interesting and personally relevant,
3. tasks completed by learners should be authentic in the sense that they allow learners to approach the concepts or the discipline in ways that a professional or an educated citizen might approach them beyond an educational programme,
4. the learning environment should be as complex as the environment of subsequent application, not a simplified version,
5. learners should be given ownership of the process for solving the problem or completing the task,
6. the learning environment should support and challenge the learners' thinking by allowing them to take the lead in puzzling through, with coaching and feedback from a tutor or instructor,

7. learners should be encouraged to test their views against alternative views and in alternative contexts,
8. instructors or tutors should support reflection by learners on the concepts learned and the process of learning, itself.

Dunlap and Grabinger offer a similar set of principles and the importance of learner autonomy is, once again, emphasized.[17] Clearly, the values of personal relevance, personal autonomy and active engagement are central to these principles which, in turn, highlight the importance of consistently harnessing learners' interest and intrinsic motivation. It may require educational designers who are sufficiently empathetic to be able to select or design problems and tasks that are very likely to engage learners' interest and sustain intrinsic motivation over time.

Several features of the ATLAS and ATHENA programmes may be regarded as engaging learners in authentic problem-solving activities relating to topics of substantial personal relevance. Both of these programmes are targeted at teenagers in high school sport teams – a social context in which the participants share common goals. They are gender-specific programmes (ATLAS for males, ATHENA for females) which may further simplify the challenge of engaging learners in problems of personal relevance. The ATLAS programme, tailored to the short-term focus of many adolescent males, focuses on the immediate effects of various substances on sport performance rather than on long term effects which may be regarded as more abstract and less engaging for the target audience. In-class activities are based on role plays and educational games, as well as the student-created public information campaign. Other programme activities take place in the gym – perhaps one place where students are likely to encounter opportunities to engage in PED use.

Nevertheless, it is not hard to conceive of improvements that might be made to these programmes. The design of credible, relevant and highly-motivating activities in a drug education programme requires empathy with the experiences of the athletes for whom the programme is intended. Research-based knowledge about the types of early encounters that young athletes tend to have with PEDs – how, when, where and with whom – would go a long way in helping educational designers to meet this challenge.

Structuring interaction among learners: more than mere 'group work'

It is not uncommon for educators and students to express frustration with what is commonly referred to as 'group work'. Free riders, coordination problems and a vague sense of 'the blind leading the blind' are common complaints. However, educational researchers have long emphasized the crucial importance of educators managing the structure of student interaction in group learning activities. Research findings on a wide range of learner interaction patterns are available including conflict or controversy, the co-construction of ideas and explanation or elaboration.[18]

The Piagetian view of socio-cognitive conflict hypothesises is that a learner who is exposed, though interaction, to ideas that differ from his or her own will experience disequilibration, forcing the learner into cognitive restructuring, via assimilation and accommodation, in search of equilibrium. Although differing views are expressed externally, the cognitive conflict occurs internally and individually. Taking this process one step further, some researchers have hypothesized that overt conflict and controversy among learners may drive internal cognitive restructuring and conceptual understanding. However, research has yielded mixed findings. Johnson and Johnson found that controversy in a group of learners can increase learning *if* learners seek additional information to resolve conflicting ideas.[19] Smith, Johnson and Johnson also found that when learners are organized into teams to prepare for a formal debate between teams, that learners improve their own understanding of concepts by reorganizing and clarifying their ideas in preparation for justifying them to others.[20] This resulted in higher achievement for those engaged in the debates versus controls. However, it should be noted that the final stage in the latter study involved the two debating teams working together to synthesize their different positions. Both of these studies illustrate an important aspect of the hypothesized effect of conflict and controversy on the development of conceptual understanding – namely that much depends on how the conflict is *resolved*.[21] It is the resolution of conflict, not the conflict *per se*, that leads to cognitive restructuring.

Other studies have been less supportive of the hypothesis that conflict promotes cognitive development. Some have reported the suppression of conflict via the domination of one or several group members, the development of group norms not to challenge others,[22] or 'pseudoconsensus' in which nonsensical or utterly relativistic conclusions are reached to avoid conflict, e.g. on a conservation task: 'When you look at it, it is bigger, but when I'm looking, they are just the same.'[23] Bearison, Magzamen and Filardo reported an inverted-U shaped relationship between conflict and cognitive gains.[24] Learners who engaged in moderate amounts of disagreement showed greater cognitive gains than learners who expressed disagreement infrequently or very frequently. They conclude that too much conflict may actually prevent group members from seeking new information to resolve their disagreements. Again, it is the resolution of conflict that leads to conceptual development.

The constructive resolution of conflict requires that some new or modified concept or explanation be negotiated by the participants. Cognitive development might not be supported by conflict *per se* but by processes of co-elaboration in which differing ideas are examined and modified to produce a new idea that takes the initial ideas into account.[25] When cooperative situations are structured appropriately, groups of learners working together may construct new ideas and principles that none of the group members could produce alone. The group constructs new or modified concepts of which all individual group members may claim ownership.

The collaborative co-construction of knowledge is at the core of Vygotskian social constructivism. Through collaboration, learners can co-construct knowledge that they did not have prior to collaboration and, through internalization, make that new knowledge their own. Research has documented positive individual learning outcomes from collaborative knowledge construction in chemistry, transformational geometry and moral reasoning.[26]

The importance of externalization or articulation in the construction of conceptual understanding is reinforced by a set of studies on peer tutoring, reciprocal teaching and reciprocal questioning.[27]

The most interesting and consistent finding of all three research programmes has been that gains in understanding are more strongly associated with the active roles of tutor, explainer or instructor than with the more passive roles of listener or learner. The act of explaining a concept to a peer encourages the explainer to clarify and restructure the concept, to generate new perspectives and to recognize gaps in his or her own understanding. Furthermore, by accommodating explanations to the difficulties of other learners, the explainer often constructs more elaborate conceptualizations for him or herself. Receiving elaborated explanations has also been hypothesized to improve a learner's conceptual understanding, but research results have consistently shown that explainers stand to gain more than receivers in terms of conceptual understanding. The types of explanations thought to be most effective for cognitive restructuring include:

- using multiple representations to explain a concept (e.g. words, diagrams, mathematical symbols),
- showing how to coordinate or translate among different representations, generating specific examples to illustrate general concepts,

- translating unfamiliar terminology into familiar terms,
- creating analogies to relate new concepts to familiar ideas,
- describing relationships between different concepts,
- using concepts to justify the reasoning used to solve a problem,
- comparing shared or personal experiences with the predictions of new concepts.[28]

Teaching and explaining are most effective for developing one's own conceptual understanding when the explanation is a genuine attempt to help another person understand the concept. This suggests the possibility that formal learner presentations may be less effective for conceptual development than informal peer teaching in smaller groups.

This is a robust finding which suggests that there may be value in having young athletes *teach* their own peers (or possibly teach younger athletes) about issues surrounding the decision to use or not to use performance-enhancing substances.

Clearly, much comes down to the careful structuring or 'scaffolding' of learner interaction. The gains in conceptual understanding that can result from interaction are not simply an automatic outcome of putting learners into groups. This, combined with the challenge of consistently harnessing the interest and intrinsic motivation of learners, suggests that designing and maintaining effective constructivist or social constructivist learning environments may be quite challenging. Furthermore, although the approach puts more responsibility for learning on to the learners themselves, substantial time and resources are required to design and maintain the learning environment. In addition, learner interaction tends to be more constructive when a tutor or facilitator works with groups of learners, so the approach can be quite demanding on human resources. Nevertheless, the cited studies show that it can be done and, if done appropriately, gains in learners' conceptual understanding can be achieved.

The ATLAS and ATHENA programmes utilize small group interaction which they attempt to structure by way of formal scripting and prior training of selected team members as facilitators. Sport team coaches also act as facilitators. However, there is no way to know how the interaction pattern actually unfolds during the programme activities or the extent to which the athletes are supportively pushed to articulate their beliefs and to challenge the espoused beliefs of others. There is a possibility that many of the athletes may simply be learning the right thing to say in the context of a drug education programme. When this possibility is combined with the research method used in the initial evaluation of these programmes – self-report questionnaires on which respondents were not anonymous – it seems that a crucial question remains unanswered: Do changes in student survey responses actually reflect changes in beliefs about PEDs or merely their compliance with what they perceive as the expected responses? Encouragingly, Elliot, Moe, Goldberg *et al.* report similar results from a more recent study using anonymous questionnaires, but the potential problem of using self-reported data remains.[29] More intensive, smaller scale studies of these programmes, using methods other than self-report questionnaires, could potentially answer this question. This is not to say that the ATLAS and ATHENA programmes do not challenge and change students beliefs about substance use – only that this question remains to be answered conclusively.

Scaffolding the art of critical enquiry: a challenging role for facilitators

Programmes that surface, challenge and reshape students' beliefs about PED use would be a fine first step in bringing the benefits of educational research and state-of-the-art educational design to bear on this issue. However, a more ambitious objective would be to equip young athletes with the skills and values to engage in this process for themselves so that they can continue to challenge and develop their own and their peers' beliefs about the topic – to build their own knowledge, autonomously, so to speak. The sociocultural approach to research on human learning is concerned with the development of individuals' capabilities for engaging in the social practices and discourses of a community of enquiry. Its educational objective is to develop, within a group, the discourse and practice of critical enquiry – to model the language and behaviour of practically-oriented *researchers*. In simple terms, this approach seeks to give students the tools and experience to approach and resolve ambiguous problems by finding out more about the problem. Although this approach is relatively new within educational design and development, there have been several well-publicized efforts to establish educational methods based on this principle.

An example from mathematics education

Greeno and his colleagues have developed an approach to mathematics pedagogy through which learners are intended to learn how to *think* mathematically and how to *become* applied mathematicians.[30] In short, learners learn how to become competent participants in the *thinking practices* used by the community of applied mathematicians. They do this by using mathematics to engage, collaboratively, with simplified versions of the realistic problems encountered by various professional users of mathematics – architectural design, logistics, modelling and simulation of natural systems, encryption or decryption of secret codes and a host of similar problems.

The research is framed by the theoretical assumption that thinking is a socially-organized practice involving reflection and discourse on activities in which we engage, and on the meanings of concepts used for planning, evaluating or making sense of those activities. In this theoretical framework, learners learn to think by participating in activities where they actively engage in thinking. In doing so, over time, they develop habits of mind or habits of thinking[31] – 'habits' being more than 'skills' in that they carry a normative weight within a practice community and may come to be valued by learners who internalize the community's norms as they begin to identify themselves with that community.

From this perspective, the practice of thinking is socially-organized via norms of enquiry, norms of discourse and norms of acceptable inference. Education should be concerned with helping learners to engage competently in practices of discourse and enquiry through which knowledge is constructed and shared. The particular practices espoused by Greeno include formulating and evaluating questions, problems, hypotheses, conjectures, evidence, examples, conclusions and arguments. Some of these practices are already included in social-constructivist pedagogies where they are regarded as effective means for mastering conceptual knowledge, but in Greeno's view these practices should, themselves, be considered central learning goals of education.

Dialogic inquiry

Another educational method based on these principles is Gordon Wells' Dialogic Inquiry.[32] According to Wells, enquiry ought to be the organizing principle of curricular activity. Enquiry begins with a real question that is a question motivated by a genuine desire to understand. The goal of enquiry is to make an explanatory artefact – a text, a diagram, a model or some other semiotic means of explaining one's view to others. It is by making an explanatory artefact for others that the learner extends his or her own understanding. The role of the instructor in such a classroom is to step out of the didactic role, to take on the role of a co-enquirer and to model an ethos of collaborative enquiry. The instructor is also the organizer and leader of the community's activities, who coaches learners in their attempts to engage in enquiry. Learners learn in a coached, cognitive apprenticeship.[33]

Students in the ATLAS programme do, in fact, make an explanatory artefact in the form of a public information campaign. However, it is not clear whether this artefact is the product of critical enquiry. Nor is it clear whether sport team coaches have the educational preparation to act as modellers of critical enquiry. If high school sport coaches are also college-educated high school teachers, then there is every possibility that they would have had the educational preparation to do so.

Modelling inquiry

The purpose of modelling inquiry is to cultivate in learners a disposition to engage in systematic inquiry about questions or topics in which one is interested. Inquiry is not just about mastering a body of information – it is also about being open to puzzlement, and trying to construct and test explanations of the phenomena that evoked these feelings.[34]

Like Greeno, Wells sees a new educational *objective* here, not merely a new educational means to an old objective. Learners are to be coached in activities of enquiry, not merely as a means of understanding prescribed theoretical concepts, but in order to prepare them to engage in practical enquiry throughout life.

Of course, not all discussion is of a type that might be expected to support the construction of valid and relevant knowledge. Hence, an important task for instructors in a programme based on Dialogic Inquiry is to actively shape the norms of discourse within the community of enquiry. An instructor should not merely supervise, but actually engage as a participant in dialogue with groups of learners to model norms for responding to statements in ways that seek to advance understanding. They should coach learners attempting to appropriate these norms. They should also lead reflective discussions to help learners articulate and evaluate the effectiveness of those norms.

The particular form of dialogue that Wells advocates is shaped by what Bereiter has termed the norms of *progressive discourse*.[35] According to both authors, a community of enquiry that upholds the norms of progressive discourse can engage in genuine knowledge building.

Knowledge Building

A third educational method incorporating the principles of critical enquiry is the Knowledge Building method of Bereiter and Scardamalia.[36] Bereiter describes the objective of this educational method as the *enculturation* of learners into the practices of a knowledge-building community.[37] Enculturation of learners into the practices of a knowledge-building community can be viewed as:

> joining the ranks of those who are familiar with, understand, create, and work with the conceptual artefacts of their culture... 'Joining the ranks' means becoming part of the knowledge-producing subculture, identifying with its members, learning their skills, sharing their aims and their norms.[38]

Bereiter's concept of Knowledge Building in education is based on the creation and improvement of conceptual artefacts (or knowledge representations) by groups of collaborating learners – a process shaped by social norms of progressive discourse.

He posits four fundamental norms underlying the progressive discourse:

1. Work toward common understanding satisfactory to all,
2. Frame questions and propositions in ways that allow evidence to be brought to bear on them,

3. Expand the body of collectively valid propositions,
4. Allow any belief to be subjected to criticism if it will advance the discourse.

When people engage in dialogue based on norms of progressive discourse, they can construct 'a new understanding that everyone involved agrees is superior to their own previous understanding'.[39]

When expressed abstractly, the objectives here may sometimes sound like the practices of scientific research. However, they are not so different from the information search, evaluation, discussion and decision making practices that are helpful to anyone when purchasing a car, taking out a mortgage, deciding who to vote for or deciding whether or not to try using PEDs. They are some of the fundamental skills needed by citizens in a democratic society and by consumers in a market economy, which is why they have found their way to the heart of the debate about what constitutes a liberal education. They could form the core of a drug education programme aimed at equipping athletes to make informed, rational decisions.

What education needs to know

The main thing we need to know is whether the constructivist educational methods, which appear to have worked successfully in formal education settings, are likely to be as effective in educating groups of athletes beyond formal education institutions. All of the educational methods discussed in this essay are based on engaging relatively small groups of peers in a workshop format, with a skilled and well-prepared instructor acting as a facilitator. Initial steps could involve small-scale design experiments, which follow a research, development and evaluation pattern.[40] Although they are labour-intensive, their small scale serves to limit the associated expense. We already have a baseline educational model in the ATLAS and ATHENA programmes. Despite the questions raised earlier, these programmes do appear to have had some degree of positive impact on young athletes. They are also consistent with a number of the design principles espoused in this essay. However, that is not to say that these programmes cannot be improved – perhaps vastly improved – by developing them further and incorporating more state-of-the-art educational techniques, such as structured interaction, peer teaching and the modelling of critical enquiry. These programmes should also be subjected to more focused, smaller-scale evaluation studies using a broader range of research methods than the self-report questionnaire. In short, we need to know what these programmes and their successors can achieve in terms of challenging and changing athletes' beliefs and equipping those athletes with the skills to locate and evaluate information and make informed decisions about the use of PEDs.

For the purpose of designing new educational programmes, it would be useful to gain an understanding of the prevailing beliefs of athletes about the use of PEDs and its consequences. Given the current lack of information about athletes' existing beliefs, it seems that a qualitative research project, based on in-depth interviews, would be an appropriate start.

It would also be useful to know more about the types of contexts in which younger athletes first encounter opportunities to try using PEDs. These are the contexts in which we want them to apply what they have learned in education programmes so the programmes themselves ought to be appropriately informed.

A research agenda for education

There are three main areas of research which would serve to augment the contribution of education towards developing a social science of drugs in sport:

1. Programme Evaluation – As the oldest form of prevention-based deterrence, more information is needed on how well these initiatives have done. For example, NADOs

often run education programmes without reporting their effect, or if they do, in terms of internal reporting functions. Achieving rigorous evaluation of education programmes to determine which approach or approaches are most effective may require input from experts experienced in such exercises. For example, this includes developing ways of identifying which parts of which programmes had more or less effect than other parts. There is also some skill involved in tracking athletes who have been exposed to educational interventions to determine the extent to which the intervention had an effect relative to other interventions (e.g. the effect of education *versus* the effect of an out-of-competition drug test).

2. Existing Knowledge – As a corollary to the first part of the agenda, more work is needed to find out just how much athletes know. Evidence that exists from bodybuilding and power lifting indicates that athletes are often very knowledgeable about the drugs they use and the risks they take.[41] If this result proves to be robust across sports, some effort needs to be made to determine whether this information influences PED use, perhaps in terms of level of processing (surface) or segregation (understood in an abstract way but has no influence on behaviour). This then feeds back into the development of more robust programmes aimed at giving athletes the capacity to process what they have learned at a deeper level.
3. Evolution of Drug Use – The final part of the agenda for education is to explore how educational effects vary over the career of the athlete. For example, the ATLAS and ATHENA programmes appear to have some effect for adolescent athletes. The question of its effect on adult athletes, perhaps in the later stages of their careers, remains unclear. While most education occurs in the pre-adult phases of life, the role of adult education also needs to be addressed. Education may also need to vary based on the longevity of career, or by sport. For example, the window of opportunity to provide effective education for Olympic-level female gymnasts is very different from that available to educate semi-professional cyclists.

It might be unwise to place too much hope on education campaigns, conducted in isolation. The potential of education, alone, to make lasting changes in human behaviour may be quite limited. However, an education programme, based on credible information, emphasizing critical inquiry and rational decision making could work in concert with other deterrence strategies by equipping athletes to make informed decisions about performance-enhancing drug use.

Notes

1 Bransford, Brown and Cocking, *How People Learn*; Greeno, Collins and Resnick, 'Cognition and Learning'.

2 Lebow, 'Constructivist Values for Systems Design', 5.

3 Donovan *et al.*, 'A Conceptual Framework for Achieving Performance Enhancing Drug Compliance in Sport'.

4 Goldberg *et al.*, 'The Adolescents Training and Learning to Avoid Steroids (ATLAS) Program'; Goldberg *et al.*, 'Effects of a Multidimensional Anabolic Steroid Prevention Intervention'; Goldberg *et al.*, 'The Adolescents Training and Learning to Avoid Steroids Program'; Elliot *et al.*, 'Preventing Substance Use and Disordered Eating', Elliott *et al.*, 'Definition and Outcome of a Curriculum to Prevent Disordered Eating and Body-shaping Drug Use'.

5 Goldberg *et al.*, 'The Adolescents Training and Learning to Avoid Steroids (ATLAS) Program'.

6 Elliot *et al.*, 'Preventing Substance Use and Disordered Eating'.

7 Durham, 'Results from the ATLAS and ATHENA Programs'.

8 Bransford, Brown and Cocking, *How People Learn*; Greeno, Collins and Resnick, 'Cognition and Learning'.

9 Bereiter and Scardamalia, 'Cognitive Coping Strategies and the Problem of Inert Knowledge'; Gabrys. Weiner and Lesgold, 'Learning by Problem Solving in a Coached Apprenticeship System'; Whitehead, *The Aims of Education.*

10 Clement, 'Student Preconceptions of Introductory Mechanics'; DiSessa, 'Unlearning Aristotelian Physics'.

11 Nesher, 'Microworlds in Mathematical Education'.

12 Piaget, *The Psychology of Intelligence*; Piaget, *The Equilibrium of Cognitive Structures.*

13 Vygotsky, *Mind in Society.*

14 Hogan and Tudge, 'Implications of Vygotsky's Theory for Peer Learning'.

15 Hatano, 'Time to Merge Vygotskian and Constructivist Conceptions of Knowledge Acquisition'; John-Steiner and Meehan, 'Creativity and Collaboration in Knowledge Construction'.

16 Dunlap and Grabinger, 'Rich Environments for Active Learning in the Higher Education Classroom'; Savery and Duffy, 'Problem Based Learning'.

17 More general treatments, along with relevant research findings, can be found in Greeno, Collins and Resnick, 'Cognition and Learning' and in the US National Research Council's report on developments in the science of human learning, Bransford, Brown and Cocking, *How People Learn.*

18 Brown and Palincsar, 'Guided, Cooperative Learning and Individual Knowledge Acquisition'; Webb and Palincsar, 'Group Processes in the Classroom'; Rogoff, 'Cognition as a Collaborative Process'.

19 Johnson and Johnson, 'Conflict in the Classroom'.

20 Smith, Johnson and Johnson, 'Effects of Controversy on Learning in Cooperative Groups'.

21 Webb and Palincsar, 'Group Processes in the Classroom'; Rogoff, 'Cognition as a Collaborative Process'.

22 Johnson and Johnson, 'Conflict in the Classroom'.

23 Brown and Palincsar, 'Guided, Cooperative Learning and Individual Knowledge Acquisition', 407.

24 Bearison, Magzamen and Filardo, 'Socio-conflict and Cognitive Growth in Young Children'.

25 Brown and Palincsar, 'Guided, Cooperative Learning and Individual Knowledge Acquisition'.

26 Webb and Palincsar, 'Group Processes in the Classroom'; Damon and Phelps, 'Critical Distinctions Among Three Methods of Peer Education'; Forman and Cazden, 'Exploring Vygotskian Perspectives in Education'; Forman, 'The Role of Peer Interaction in the Social Construction of Mathematical Knowledge'; Damon and Killen, 'Peer Interaction and the Process of Change in Children's Moral Reasoning'.

27 Webb, 'Peer Interaction and Learning in Small Groups'; Webb, 'Task-related Verbal Interaction and Mathematics Learning in Small Groups'; Palincsar and Brown, 'Reciprocal Teaching of Comprehension-fostering and Comprehension-monitoring Activities'; Palincsar and Brown, 'Reciprocal Teaching: Activities to Promote "Reading with your Mind"'; Palincsar and Brown, 'Interactive Teaching to Promote Independent Learning from Text'; Brown and Palincsar, 'Guided, Cooperative Learning and Individual Knowledge Acquisition'; Brown and Campione, 'Communities of Learning and Thinking'; Brown and Campione, 'Guided Discovery in a Community of Learners'; King, 'Enhancing Peer Interaction and Learning in the Classroom'; King, 'Facilitating Elaborated Learning through Guided Student-generated Questioning'; King, 'Guiding Knowledge Construction in the Classroom'; King, 'Discourse Patterns for Mediating Peer Learning'.

28 Webb and Palincsar, 'Group Processes in the Classroom'.

29 Elliott *et al.*, 'Definition and Outcome of a Curriculum to Prevent Disordered Eating and Body-shaping Drug Use'.

30 Greeno *et al.*, 'Theories and Practices of Thinking and Learning to Think'.

31 Dewey, *Democracy and Education.*

32 Wells, *Dialogic Inquiry*; Wells, 'Dialogic Inquiry in the Classroom'; Wells, 'Dialogue about Knowledge Building'.

33 Collins, 'Cognitive Apprenticeship and Instructional Technology'; Collins, Brown and Newman, 'Cognitive Apprenticeship'.

34 Wells, 'Dialogic Inquiry in the Classroom'.

35 Bereiter, 'Implications of Postmodernism for Science'.

36 Bereiter, 'Situated Cognition and How to Overcome It'; Bereiter, 'Liberal Education in a Knowledge Society'; Bereiter, 'Artifacts, Canons and the Progress of Pedagogy'; Bereiter and Scardamalia, 'Rethinking Learning'; Bereiter and Scardamalia, 'Beyond Bloom's Taxonomy'; Bereiter and Scardamalia, 'Commentary on Part I'; Scardamalia, 'Collective Cognitive Responsibility for the Advancement of Knowledge'; Scardamalia and Bereiter, 'Engaging Students in a Knowledge Society'; Scardamalia, Bereiter and Lamon, 'The CSILE Project'.

37 Bereiter, 'Artifacts, Canons and the Progress of Pedagogy'.
38 Ibid., 229.
39 Bereiter, 'Implications of Postmodernism for Science', 6.
40 Brown, 'Design Experiments'; Collins, 'Toward a Design Science of Education'.
41 Grogan *et al.*, 'Experience of Anabolic Steroid Use'.

References

Bearison, D.J., S. Magzamen, and E.K. Filardo. 'Socio-conflict and Cognitive Growth in Young Children'. *Merrill-Palmer Quarterly* 32 (1986): 51–72.

Bereiter, C. 'Implications of Postmodernism for Science, or, Science as Progressive Discourse'. *Educational Psychologist* 29, no. 1 (1994): 3–12.

Bereiter, C. 'Situated Cognition and How to Overcome It'. In *Situated Cognition: Social, Semiotic and Psychological Perspectives*, edited by D. Kirshner and J.A. Whitson, 281–300. Mahwah, NJ: Lawrence Erlbaum, 1997.

Bereiter, C. 'Liberal Education in a Knowledge Society'. In *Liberal Education in a Knowledge Society*, edited by B. Smith, 11–34. Chicago, IL: Open Court, 2002.

Bereiter, C. 'Artifacts, Canons and the Progress of Pedagogy: A Response to Contributors'. In *Liberal Education in a Knowledge Society*, edited by B. Smith, 223–44. Chicago, IL: Open Court, 2002.

Bereiter, C., and M. Scardamalia. 'Cognitive Coping Strategies and the Problem of Inert Knowledge'. In *Thinking and Learning Skills: Current Research and Open Questions*, edited by S.F. Chipman, J.W. Segal, and R. Glaser, 65–80. Hillsdale, NJ: Lawrence Erlbaum, 1985.

Bereiter, C., and M. Scardamalia. 'Rethinking Learning'. In *The Handbook of Education and Human Development: New Models of Learning, Teaching and Schooling*, edited by D.R. Olson and N. Torrance, 485–513. Cambridge, MA: Blackwell, 1996.

Bereiter, C., and M. Scardamalia. 'Beyond Bloom's Taxonomy: Rethinking Knowledge for the Knowledge Age'. In *International Handbook of Educational Change*, edited by A. Hargreaves, A. Liebermann, M. Fullan, and D. Hopkins, 675–92. Boston, MA: Kluwer, 1998.

Bereiter, C., and M. Scardamalia. 'Commentary on Part I: Process and Product in Problem-based Learning Research'. In *Problem-based Learning: A Research Perspective on Learning Interactions*, edited by D.H. Evensen and C.E. Hmelo, 185–98. Mahwah, NJ: Lawrence Erlbaum, 2000.

Bransford, J.D., A.L. Brown, and R.R. Cocking, eds. *How People Learn: Brain, Mind, Experience and School*. Washington, DC: National Academy Press, 2001.

Brown, A.L. 'Design Experiments: Theoretical and Methodological Challenges in Creating Complex Interventions'. *Journal of Learning Sciences* 2, no. 2 (1992): 141–78.

Brown, A.L., and J.C. Campione. 'Communities of Learning and Thinking, or a Context by Any Other Name'. *Developmental Perspectives on Learning and Teaching Thinking Skills* 21 (1990): 108–26.

Brown, A.L., and J.C. Campione. 'Guided Discovery in a Community of Learners'. In *Classroom Lessons: Integrating Cognitive Theory and Classroom Practice*, edited by K. McGilly, 229–70. Cambridge, MA: MIT Press, 1994.

Brown, A.L., and A.S. Palincsar. 'Guided, Cooperative Learning and Individual Knowledge Acquisition'. In *Knowing, Learning and Instruction: Essays in Honor of Robert Glaser*, edited by L.B. Resnick, 393–408. Hillsdale, NJ: Lawrence Erlbaum Associates, 1989.

Clement, J. 'Student Preconceptions of Introductory Mechanics'. *American Journal of Physics* 50 (1982): 66–71.

Collins, A. 'Cognitive Apprenticeship and Instructional Technology'. In *Educational Values and Cognitive Instruction: Implications for Reform*, edited by L. Idol and B.F. Jones, 121–38. Hillsdale, NJ: Lawrence Erlbaum, 1991.

Collins, A. 'Toward a Design Science of Education'. In *New Directions in Educational Technology*, edited by E. Scanlon and T. O'Shea, 15–22. New York: Springer-Verlag, 1992.

Collins, A., J.S. Brown, and S.E. Newman. 'Cognitive Apprenticeship: Teaching the Crafts of Reading, Writing and Mathematics'. In *Knowing, Learning and Instruction: Essays in Honor of Robert Glaser*, edited by L.B. Resnick, 453–94. Hillsdale, NJ: Lawrence Erlbaum, 1989.

Damon, W., and M. Killen. 'Peer Interaction and the Process of Change in Children's Moral Reasoning'. *Merrill-Palmer Quarterly* 28 (1982): 347–67.

Damon, W., and E. Phelps. 'Critical Distinctions Among Three Methods of Peer Education'. *International Journal of Educational Research* 13 (1989): 9–19.

Dewey, J. *Democracy and Education: An Introduction to the Philosophy of Education*. New York: Macmillan, 1916.

DiSessa, A. 'Unlearning Aristotelian Physics. A Study of Knowledge-based Learning'. *Cognitive Science* 6 (1982): 37–75.

Donovan, R.J., G. Egger, V. Kapernick, and J. Mendoza. 'A Conceptual Framework for Achieving Performance Enhancing Drug Compliance in Sport'. *Sports Medicine* 32, no. 4 (2002): 269–84.

Dunlap, J.C., and R.S. Grabinger. 'Rich Environments for Active Learning in the Higher Education Classroom'. In *Constructivist Learning Environments: Case Studies in Instructional Design*, edited by B.G. Wilson, 65–82. Englewood Cliffs, NJ: Educational Testing Publications, 1996.

Durham, M. 'Results from the ATLAS and ATHENA Programs'. Paper presented at the WADA Conference Ethics and Social Science Research in Anti-doping, Larnaca, Cyprus, April 13–14, 2006.

Elliot, D.L., L. Goldberg, E.L. Moe, C.A. DeFrancesco, M.B. Durham, and H. Hix-Small. 'Preventing Substance Use and Disordered Eating: Initial Outcomes of the ATHENA (Athletes Targeting Healthy Exercise and Nutrition Alternatives) Program'. *Archives of Pediatrics and Adolescent Medicine* 158 (2004): 1043–9.

Elliott, D.L., E.L. Moe, L. Goldberg, C.A. DeFrancesco, M.B. Durham, and H. Hix-Small. 'Definition and Outcome of a Curriculum to Prevent Disordered Eating and Body-shaping Drug Use'. *Journal of School Health* 76, no. 2 (2006): 67–73.

Forman, E.A. 'The Role of Peer Interaction in the Social Construction of Mathematical Knowledge'. *International Journal of Educational Research* 13 (1989): 55–70.

Forman, E.A., and C.B. Cazden. 'Exploring Vygotskian Perspectives in Education: The Cognitive Value of Peer Interaction'. In *Culture, Communication and Cognition: Vygotskian Perspectives*, edited by J.V. Wertsch, 323–47. New York, NY: Cambridge University Press, 1985.

Gabrys, G., A. Weiner, and A. Lesgold. 'Learning by Problem Solving in a Coached Apprenticeship System'. In *Cognitive Science Foundations of Instruction*, edited by M. Rabinowitz, 119–47. Hillsdale, NJ: Lawrence Erlbaum, 1993.

Goldberg, L., D.L. Elliot, G.N. Clarke, D.P. MacKinnon, L. Zoref, E. Moe, C. Green, and S.L. Wolf. 'The Adolescents Training and Learning to Avoid Steroids (ATLAS) Program: Background and Results of a Model Intervention'. *Archives of Pediatrics and Adolescent Medicine* 150, no. 7 (1996): 713–21.

Goldberg, L., D.L. Elliot, G.N. Clarke, D.P. MacKinnon, L. Zoref, E. Moe, C. Green, S.L. Wolf, E. Greffrath, D.J. Miller, and A. Lapin. 'Effects of a Multidimensional Anabolic Steroid Prevention Intervention: The Adolescents Training and Learning to Avoid Steroids (ATLAS) Program'. *JAMA: Journal of the American Medical Association* 276, no. 19 (1996): 1555–62.

Goldberg, L., D.P. MacKinnon, D.L. Elliot, E.L. Moe, G. Clarke, and J. Cheong. 'The Adolescents Training and Learning to Avoid Steroids Program: Preventing Drug Use and Promoting Health Behaviors'. *Archives of Pediatrics and Adolescent Medicine* 154 (2000): 332–8.

Greeno, J.G., A.M. Collins, and L.B. Resnick. 'Cognition and Learning'. In *Handbook of Educational Psychology*, edited by D.C. Berliner and R.C. Calfee, 15–46. New York: Macmillan, 1996.

Greeno, J.G. and The Middle-School Mathematics Through Applications Project Group. 'Theories and Practices of Thinking and Learning to Think'. *American Journal of Education* 106, no. 1 (1997): 85–126.

Grogan, S., S. Shepherd, R. Evans, S. Wright, and G. Hunter. 'Experience of Anabolic Steroid Use: In-depth Interviews with Men and Women Body Builders'. *Journal of Health Psychology* 11 (2006): 845–56.

Hatano, G. 'Time to Merge Vygotskian and Constructivist Conceptions of Knowledge Acquisition'. In *Contexts for Learning: Sociocultural Dynamics in Children's Development*, edited by E.A. Forman, N. Minnick, and C.A. Stone, 153–66. New York: Oxford University Press, 1993.

Hogan, D.M., and J.R.H. Tudge. 'Implications of Vygotsky's Theory for Peer Learning'. In *Cognitive Perspectives on Peer Learning*, edited by A.M. O'Donnell and A. King, 39–65. Mahwah, NJ: Lawrence Erlbaum Associates, 1999.

John-Steiner, V.P., and T.M. Meehan. 'Creativity and Collaboration in Knowledge Construction'. In *Vygotskian Perspectives on Literacy Research: Constructing Meaning through Collaborative Inquiry*, edited by C.D. Lee and P. Smagorinsky, 31–50. Cambridge: Cambridge University Press, 2000.

Johnson, D.W., and R.T. Johnson. 'Conflict in the Classroom: Controversy and Learning'. *Review of Educational Research* 49 (1979): 51–70.

King, A. 'Enhancing Peer Interaction and Learning in the Classroom through Reciprocal Questioning'. *American Educational Research Journal* 27 (1990): 664–87.

King, A. 'Facilitating Elaborated Learning through Guided Student-generated Questioning'. *Educational Psychologist* 27 (1992): 111–26.

King, A. 'Guiding Knowledge Construction in the Classroom: Effects of Teaching Children How to Question and How to Explain'. *American Educational Research Journal* 31 (1994): 338–68.
King, A. 'Discourse Patterns for Mediating Peer Learning'. In *Cognitive Perspectives on Peer Learning*, edited by A.M. O'Donnell and A. King, 87–115. Mahwah, NJ: Lawrence Erlbaum Associates, 1999.
Lebow, D. 'Constructivist Values for Systems Design: Five Principles toward a New Mindset'. *Educational Technology Research and Development* 41 (1993): 4–16.
Nesher, P. 'Microworlds in Mathematical Education: A Pedagogical Realism'. In *Knowing, Learning and Instruction: Essays in Honor of Robert Glaser*, edited by L.B. Resnick, 187–216. Hillsdale, NJ: Lawrence Erlbaum, 1989.
Palincsar, A.S., and A.L. Brown. 'Reciprocal Teaching of Comprehension-fostering and Comprehension-monitoring Activities'. *Cognition and Instruction* 1 (1984): 117–75.
Palincsar, A.S., and A.L. Brown. 'Reciprocal Teaching: Activities to Promote "Reading with your Mind"'. In *Reading, Thinking and Concept Development: Interactive Strategies for the Class*, edited by E.J. Cooper, 147–58. New York: College Board, 1985.
Palincsar, A.S., and A.L. Brown. 'Interactive Teaching to Promote Independent Learning from Text'. *The Reading Teacher* 39, no. 8 (1986): 771–7.
Piaget, J. *The Psychology of Intelligence*. Totowa, NJ: Littlefield, Adams and Co, 1966.
Piaget, J. *The Equilibrium of Cognitive Structures: The Central Problem of Intellectual Development*. Chicago, IL: University of Chicago Press, 1985.
Rogoff, B. 'Cognition as a Collaborative Process'. In *Handbook of Child Development. Volume 2: Cognition, Perception and Language*, edited by D. Kuhn and R.S. Siegler, 679–744. New York: John Wiley and Sons, 1998.
Savery, J.R., and T.M. Duffy. 'Problem Based Learning: An Instructional Model and its Constructivist Framework'. In *Constructivist Learning Environments: Case Studies in Instructional Design*, edited by B.G. Wilson. Englewood Cliffs, NJ: Educational Testing Publications, 1996.
Scardamalia, M. 'Collective Cognitive Responsibility for the Advancement of Knowledge'. In *Liberal Education in a Knowledge Society*, edited by B. Smith, 67–98. Chicago, IL: Open Court, 2002.
Scardamalia, M., and C. Bereiter. 'Engaging Students in a Knowledge Society'. *Educational Leadership* 54, no. 3 (1996): 6–10.
Scardamalia, M., C. Bereiter, and M. Lamon. 'The CSILE Project: Trying to Bring the Classroom into World 3'. In *Classroom Lessons: Integrating Cognitive Theory and Classroom Practice*, edited by K. McGilly, 201–28. Cambridge, MA: MIT Press, 1994.
Smith, K., D.W. Johnson, and R.T. Johnson. 'Effects of Controversy on Learning in Cooperative Groups'. *Journal of Social Psychology* 122 (1984): 199–209.
Vygotsky, L.S. *Mind in Society: The Development of Higher Psychological Processes*. Cambridge, MA: Harvard University Press, 1978.
Webb, N.M. 'Peer Interaction and Learning in Small Groups'. *International Journal of Educational Research* 13 (1989): 21–40.
Webb, N.M. 'Task-related Verbal Interaction and Mathematics Learning in Small Groups'. *Journal for Research into Mathematics Education* 22 (1991): 366–89.
Webb, N.M., and A.S. Palincsar. 'Group Processes in the Classroom'. In *Handbook of Educational Psychology*, edited by D. Berliner and R. Calfee, 841–73. New York: Macmillan, 1996.
Wells, G. *Dialogic Inquiry: Towards a Sociocultural Practice and Theory of Education*. Cambridge: Cambridge University Press, 1999.
Wells, G. 'Dialogic Inquiry in the Classroom: Building on the Legacy of Vygotsky'. In *Vygotskian Perspectives on Literacy Research*, edited by C. Lee and P. Smagorinsky, 51–85. New York: Cambridge University Press, 2000.
Wells, G. 'Dialogue about Knowledge Building'. In *Liberal Education in a Knowledge Society*, edited by B. Smith, 111–38. Chicago, IL: Open Court, 2002.
Whitehead, A.N. *The Aims of Education*. Cambridge: Cambridge University Press, 1929.

Without bounds: A cosmopolitan research agenda for drugs in sport

Jason Mazanov

School of Business, UNSW@ADFA, Canberra, Australia

The role of 'cosmopolitan research' was considered as a key platform with which to build a social science of drugs in sport. Cosmopolitan research is characterized as explaining human behaviour without regard for disciplinary boundaries, defined through questions that can be approached by any discipline and responded to by, preferably, collaboration across the disciplines. Three such questions are posed and explored to identify areas for collaborative research. The contributions from across the collection examining social science and drugs in sport research are analysed and synthesized to establish common areas for future research. Based on these questions and common themes, an agenda for cosmopolitan research into drugs in sport phenomena is articulated.

Where examination of the drugs in sport literature identifies very little in the way of social science based research,[1] there is even less that makes use of inter-disciplinary approaches. This essay combines the research ideas and results from discipline specific perspectives (from across the collection) to establish a set of novel or innovative collaborative drugs in sport research projects. The desire to innovate towards collaborative research was a feature of the way contributors to the current collection approached the project.

This essay explores cosmopolitan rather than multidisciplinary research. To explain the difference between cosmopolitan and multidisciplinary research, the analogy of the 'Individual, Group and Organization' is offered. Social science is reconceptualized as an organization ('Social Science Incorporated') whose primary business is to resolve questions about and understand human behaviour in its many forms. The group level is represented by the different disciplines, each seeking to achieve Social Science Inc.'s purpose using different ways of thinking (philosophies) and different methods (such as statistical tools). Quite often this means exploring or explaining the same thing using different language (the jargon of a specific discipline), emphasizing one pattern of results over another, or providing a very different interpretation for the same pattern of results. The individual level is then represented by the people working in each group; for example psychology can be interpreted from several different perspectives (e.g. health and educational). Each 'individual' uses a highly specialized way of deducing explanations about how the world works.

The individual sub-disciplines learn a lot about human behaviour from their particular perspective, which comes together to form the disciplinary or group understanding of human behaviour. When the disciplines come together they might look for multidisciplinary explanations of human behaviour, where results complement each other or they discover they have explained the same thing in different ways; easy in theory and very difficult in practice. Where multidisciplinary explanations emerge, these ideas go into the mix at the organizational level where the executive management of Social Science Inc. start explaining human behaviour; importantly, they do so without regard for disciplinary boundaries. These aggregate explanations of human behaviour achieve the main business of Social Science Inc.[2] It is at this organizational or 'executive' level of social science that cosmopolitan research emerges. That is, cosmopolitan research is interested in explaining human behaviour without regard for disciplinary boundaries. This cosmopolitan approach also means asking questions that have similar disregard for disciplinary boundaries; asking questions to which any discipline can contribute. For example, instead of asking about how psychology or a combination of psychology and economics predicts prohibited performance-enhancing substances or methods (PESM) use by athletes, the cosmopolitan question asks 'what makes an athlete use prohibited PESM?'

Cosmopolitan research, as defined here, has two key characteristics. The first is the asking of general questions that can be approached by any discipline. The second is that cosmopolitan research scans across the disciplines to identify areas of common interest that might usefully lead to effective collaboration across the disciplines.[3] This is how this essay is structured. The first section reports the results of a workshop on social science and drugs in sport (July 2006). The World Café method was employed to develop questions about drugs in sport intended to stimulate interest from across the social science disciplines. The second section reports on areas of common interest that emerge from an analysis of the discipline specific contributions to this collection, categorized into three themes that represent questions deserving of further investigation by any diverse research team (either as organized research teams, through the literature, through policy, over the internet, or over coffee).

The second World Café

The World Café method asks contributors to come up with a range of questions worthy of consideration. Once the requisite number of questions have been achieved (in this case three), the conversation around each question is hosted by one person and joined by several discussants. The host's job is to introduce the topic and invite people to participate in the discussion. After a period of time (about 45 minutes) the discussants change tables to examine a new issue, while the host remains to introduce the question again. Continuity is achieved through the host, and all the disciplines can interact through this continuity. This means ensuring each discipline represented at the workshop worked with each of the other disciplines across all of the questions. The following three questions were chosen by the participants for the World Café:

1. What are the public perceptions of drugs in sport issues? (hosted by Alannah Kazlauskas)
2. Are the anti-doping rules effective? (hosted by Trevor O'Donnell)
3. What is the system around drugs in sport? (hosted by Vanessa McDermott)

What are the public perceptions of drugs in sport issues?

This issue came out of vibrant debate driven by Dr James Connor (a contributor) and Professor Brian Stoddart, the latter invited to the second workshop as a recognized authority on sport sociology and sport history. The issue seemed to be a challenge to the assumption that the anti-doping stance was taken from the sport-consuming public's negative perception of drug users in sport. This is reflected in the assumption that spectators would abandon sports tainted by the use of prohibited PESM. The team could only find evidence to refute this particular assumption.[4] For example, commentators indicate PESM scandals made no obvious difference to ongoing fan support for at least American baseball and the Tour de France.[5] This led to speculation about the very general question of what the public actually thinks about drugs in sport issues. The answer to this question has implications for the anti-doping stance.

For example, if the public's view is one where they would prefer the spectacle of human performance[6] it may provoke media and gambling interests to take a different view on the use of PESM in sport. This could lead to a stance promoting management of drugs in sport aimed at helping athletes to use PESM without compromising their health.[7]

The cosmopolitan component to this question lies in its focus on public attitudes towards drugs in sport. Attitudes take many forms across social science disciplines, from the classic definitions used by psychology and sociology, to discussions of utility in economics. The sport philosopher on the team introduced the idea that the exploration of attitude in this way could be better served by thinking in terms of 'discourses'. That is, looking to the language used by people to promote, marginalize or stigmatize different ways of thinking about drugs in sport. The legal, economic, sociological and psychological approaches to drugs in sport can be very different in their use of language, or discourse, to explore the issues at hand. Add to these the medical and political discourses and this becomes an issue of finding out how people think about drugs in sport. This is a sound basic question for social science to interrogate.[8]

The educational psychologist on the team, Dr James Hanson, pointed out that people can hold multiple conflicting beliefs (attitudes) or knowledge towards a particular issue, with each one affecting behaviour at different times. For example, some one with a strong zero-tolerance towards drugs conviction may then pay for flights and accommodation to see the Tour de France because of their passion for cycling spectacle. The implication of this point is that research on public attitudes needs to find out about the multiple simultaneous beliefs held about drugs in sport issues. Research on this issue draws on an important basic question of interest to social science, the relationship between attitude and behaviour.

Conducting research into the relationship between attitude and behaviour requires a significant effort from across the social sciences. In the first instance, some serious work is needed on the different discourses associated with drugs in sport to give some indication about how people think about drugs in sport. This work defines a series of models from which questions can be developed to probe how the different discourses are represented by different people. The discourses could be promoted by different groups of people. Looking for differences between groups means thinking long and hard about where meaningful differences may lie. Further, looking at discourses across different sports may help identify why sports like cycling or weightlifting appear to be more vulnerable to prohibited PESM use. The other groups of interest are spectators, support staff, athlete peer group, gamblers, the media, academics, SGBs and NADOs.

The programme for this line of research would be well served by any one of three approaches. The first is likely to be a thorough analysis of existing discourse across media (e.g. web commentaries, annual reports and NADO campaigns). This discourse can then feed into the second approach, which would be qualitative data collection by talking to people in the groups of interest. The final approach is quantitative data collection. The normal approaches to attitude measurement use Likert-type scales (e.g. strongly agree to strongly disagree). There are other innovative ways of measuring attitude[9] such as implicit attitude measurement, dynamical modelling of attitudes, or best-worst scaling that might be useful in the drugs in sport context. The primary, qualitative and quantitative avenues for researching this question could be done sequentially, simultaneously and/or independently.

Are the anti-doping rules effective?

This question arose from a desire to gather evidence that validated or invalidated the anti-doping approach as the best way to manage drugs in sport. In looking at this issue, it is important to keep in mind that it is relatively easier to be critical of an existing system than proposing an alternative. With this in mind, the first part of the conversation concentrated on finding alternatives to anti-doping before exploring issues confronting implementation of managing drugs in sport in a policy neutral way. Talking about the question this way gave a 'future' orientation of striving towards ways of promoting more mature and evolved ways of managing drugs in sport. This mental model was used analyse the question by first looking at 'the rules' and second what might be meant by 'effective'.

The rules

The anti-doping approach is only one way of managing drugs in sport that aligns with the professed ideology of sport and pre-existing national drug management strategies (e.g. zero tolerance policies). While no system will ever be perfect, it is appropriate to ask whether the one we have is suitable for its purpose. A number of strategies to manage drugs in sport have been offered based around varying levels of permissiveness. At the extreme of prohibition no performance-enhancing substance or method would be permitted, possibly including supplements, certain training methods and so on. In the middle is the current mixed system with some permission (e.g. caffeine) and some prohibition. At the extreme of permissiveness, some commentators advocate for the removal of all management.[10] A moderate permissive position is suggested by Bird and Wagner[11] who propose athletes record all the drugs they use in a 'drug diary', with a violation and consequent sanction occurring where testing finds a performance-enhancing substance absent from the diary. Savulescu *et al.*[12] argue that drugs in sport should be managed by sanctioning athletes who engage in health-threatening drug use. For example, a positive for an EPO user would be exceeding the medically established 'safe' packed cell volume count (too many red blood cells) resulting in exclusion from competition until the count returned to the safe level.[13] This short set of examples gives some options to test which approach is likely to be the most effective in terms of managing drugs in sport relative to the desired outcomes (e.g. the Olympic ideal, health or advertising revenues).

A nagging issue that emerged from this was whether any particular approach would be sustainable over time. This reinforces the need to explore alternative approaches to drugs in sport that might cater for other changes in technology. Miah[14] has begun to travel this road with an exploration of how gene doping might influence sport and ways in which it could be managed now and in the future. It might be worthwhile testing how nanotechnology used for improving human physical capabilities[15] would be managed using any of the approaches offered here.

Effective

As part of the assessment of alternative approaches to managing drugs in sport, the team started questioning what was meant by effective.[16] The main confusion extended from the absence of a clear consensus as to the desired outcome in relation to drugs in sport policies. Miah argues that the premises underpinning anti-doping are based on highly contested terms, resulting in ambiguity as to the desired outcomes.[17] The consequence to the ambiguity is a potential failure to translate the policy intent of anti-doping championed by WADA into policy implementation at the local level;[18] that is, minimizing the number of athletes using PESMs at all of the elite, professional, semi-professional, amateur and recreational levels.

The discussants were concerned that a sound philosophy or justification was needed to establish the anti-doping stance unequivocally. If none could be found, then it should be replaced. This challenges whether the principles outlined in the WADC are good ones upon which to base a universal policy for managing drugs in sport. Some discussants were concerned that the economic or political interests of the broader sports industry (including government) interfered with the anti-doping ideology, making it a public relations exercise rather than a genuine attempt to make a stand against drugs in sport. (There was a sense that anti-doping might be more successful if industry interests were more explicitly recognized.) The discussion made it readily apparent that proponents of anti-doping need to develop a much stronger case for their stance that leads to tangible (measurable) outcomes that can be used as a basis to judge whether a policy has been effective.

A consistent theme throughout the discussion was the problem of how to measure effectiveness of any approach to managing drugs in sport. The basic question relates to how one would determine whether the approach was working (programme evaluation). A distinct hurdle is the absence of a reliable measure for prevalence of drug use in sport. Getting an indication of prevalence allows some indication of the success associated with both detection- and prevention-based deterrence, such as declining prevalence due to better targeting of detection or more effective education programmes. Another aspect of programme evaluation is Plato's question, 'who is watching the watchers?' In this case, it returns to the question of whose interests the programme serves. For example, governments may establish NADOs to ensure access to IOC funding and events (a compliance argument). This makes measures of compliance with WADA more important than prevalence rates or athlete health. Likewise, anti-doping activity in SGBs might be evaluated in terms of impact on advertising revenue rather than athlete health or well-being.[19]

Researching this question

Speculating how this line of research might be furthered involves significant collaboration between the disciplines. A key concern is resolving the issue of clarity in ideology for managing drugs in sport and what that ideology seeks to achieve (outcomes). With certainty arising from clear objectives, some assessment can be made as to what form of framework is best placed to achieve the desired outcome. This framework could usefully incorporate the role of the institution (the broader sports industry including the IOC, NADOs, governments, media and sports manufacturers) and the group (such as support staff) in relation to drugs in sport, extending the management of drugs in sport beyond policing individuals.

What is the system around drugs in sport?

The thrust of this conversation was an evaluation of the anti-doping system as it stood at the beginning of the twenty-first century. Describing the system this way achieves two goals common to all the disciplines of social science. The first is that research into the prevailing system is another avenue to understand how societies interact to solve social problems; an exploration of the human condition. To this extent there was some overlap with the previous conversation. The second was to:

- plant a flag in the ground to identify the system as it was (a benchmark) and build the opportunity to see what needs to change,
- identify how those changes might be wrought, and
- use the benchmark to measure the evolution of the prevailing drugs in sport system into something else.

Getting a sense of where the anti-doping system relies on developing accurate histories of how the system evolved. There are many histories on the role of drugs in sport from NADOs, academics and journalists. There are also histories of the institutions, such as the chain of events that led to the Lausanne Declaration and the formation of WADA. There are also histories of specific incidents, such as the development of the test for EPO.[20] What is conspicuously absent from these histories are the thoughts and comments of the architects of the system. That is, those people behind the scenes that pioneered anti-doping in terms of policy development and implementation. Constructing an oral history of anti-doping might include talking with the politicians who oversaw the introduction of anti-doping in their country, the foundation members of the laboratories that came to be WADA accredited and the foundation members of NADOs. The history could be extended to talk to those administrators who implemented the anti-doping policy 'on the ground', such as managers of sports academies, doping control officers and, of course, the athletes who experienced the system.

The host of this Café conversation, Vanessa McDermott, introduced the idea of thinking about the stakeholders involved in anti-doping and where the athlete fits in. Vanessa's subsequent speculation suggested that the athlete plays a fairly minor role compared to the bureaucracy that administers anti-doping.[21] This suggests that it is important to consider how the athletes see themselves positioned within an anti-doping system. For example, it would be valuable for the integrity and legitimacy of anti-doping[22] to take stock of whether athletes see themselves as a valued and integral part of addressing PESMs in sport. In considering the role of the athlete within the system, the team also brought up the issue of trust in the system. For example, anti-doping is so complicated that athletes are left with no alternative but to trust 'experts' in terms of PESM use (e.g. NADOs, sports physicians or coaches). Exploring the role of trust was seen as an important element to understanding the athlete's experience of the anti-doping system.

At this point, overlap began emerging with the previous Café conversation, as the discussants grappled with the institutional interactions that support the anti-doping system. One key concern was the duty of care for the public and private sectors. The private sports industry (such as the IOC, individual sports clubs and sport equipment manufacturers) rely on the public sector (in this case the government and community sectors) to support the anti-doping stance. For example, most NADOs are majority funded by taxpayers to provide services like administration of drug testing (sometimes on a fee for service basis), education and funding research. Government is also required to monitor and manage drugs in sport through the judiciary, police and customs. While it is clear the public sector is doing its best to maintain the social value of sport through anti-doping, it raises the unsettling question of what the private sector is doing. In pure financial terms, it might be interesting to find out the value private sporting organizations place on anti-doping activities by looking at much they spend on anti-doping relative to other interventions (e.g. interventions to reduce alcohol abuse or anti-social behaviour).

A big question for social science is how structures encourage or restrict behaviour. The team took a slightly different approach to the issue of structure, encouraging or restricting behaviour by questioning how the system around drugs in sport promotes innovation within the system. The basic model followed Kerr's observation that actors often reward behaviours that they hope will lead to the behaviour they want (rewarding A while hoping for B).[23] The current system seems to support the development of PESM, creative use of masking agents and detection methods. There is also systemic support for social science research projects like this one (funded by the Australian Anti-Doping Research Program) in an effort to develop innovative approaches to research drugs in sport. A barrier to innovation of the drugs in sport system lies in the administration of drugs in sport policy which is arguably an extension of the policy stance taken in the 1960s. Examining the drugs in sport system offers social science an opportunity to look at how technological innovation has been encouraged (drugs and drug testing) and perhaps how administrative innovation has been restricted.

Outcomes of the World Café

The conversations that made up the World Café inspired some different ways of thinking about drugs in sport. The theme that emerged from across the conversations was that taking a 'cosmopolitan' approach leads to questions about how the individual, group, organization and system interact to influence human behaviour.

Areas of commonality

Making sense of the combined and varied contributions in terms of commonalities that informed the cosmopolitan research agenda was challenging. The primary thematic content analysis was conducted across the contributions and included the ideas emerging from the World Café outlined above. This analysis led to two robust ideas that could be usefully explored by social science, and one that could be used to guide the practice of social science on this issue.

Performance enhancement behaviour

One of the themes emerging from across the collection pointed directly towards developing the understanding of how the 'desire to perform' influences behaviour. Responding to the use of PESM in sport identifies that more work is needed on the social science of performance enhancement; drugs in sport represents only one way in which humans seek to augment themselves technologically.[24] It may well be that the principles driving PESM use in sport also drive desires to wear expensive jewellery, be associated with socially desirable brands, submit to cosmetic surgery, or even be ambitious at work. Armed with a social science of performance enhancement it may then be possible to examine triggers for compliance and non-compliance in relation to performance within a structured, rule-driven system. For example, such a social science of performance enhancement could be applied to rule breaking among directors or board members of a company to maximize the performance of their company (e.g. share price).[25]

The methods for investigating the individual response to performance enhancement have a strong foundation in psychological science. Developing a psychology of performance enhancement fits under the umbrella of performance psychology. Work on cheating behaviour[26] might inform the tipping point to rule breaking for some desired performance-related outcome. The performance aspect might also be investigated using Game Theory to get a sense of how rational actors approach performance, especially how such actors trade off various performance outcomes relative to risks. A further component may be to gauge how individual responses (such as utilities) vary in response to different rule structures (e.g. strict liability).

The networked athlete

Girginov observed that 'manufacturing' elite athletes is an industry.[27] Each elite athlete is overseen by a project team which delivers highly specialized resources (e.g. nutrition, accommodation, training facilities, support staff, education and salary) through their management of a sophisticated organisational structure.[28] The immediate implication of this observation is that understanding the use of PESM by any athlete requires an understanding of the social networks surrounding the athlete.[29] Looking at the individual level, this means the people proximal to the athlete. The next step is going from the proximal to the distal, and having a look at who the project team interact with. That is, exploring the effects that individuals who interact only indirectly with a target athlete have on that target athlete's PESM use. At this basic level there is scope to engage in social network analysis to gain a sense of how the (elite) athlete fits into the project team. This represents only the tip of the iceberg, as a greater understanding of the relationship between parts is required, that is, the role of the athlete in the immediate social network and the broader network of groups and organizations within which they interact. Examination of the athlete's network then provides the opportunity to explore what those other groups or organizations do and their relationship with each other. That is, a stakeholder analysis of drugs in sport.

As noted above, social network analysis is one method that may help deliver results useful towards a social science of drugs in sport. What may also be useful is an in-depth examination of WADAs attempt to harmonize anti-doping efforts around the world. Creating a universal system of administering a global issue is ambitious. For example, at the time of writing harmonization on pressing issues such as climate change or biodiversity appeared to be a long way off.[30] Houlihan[31] has documented anti-doping's efforts towards harmonization and its implications as a case study, offering a solid and grounded launching point from which other researchers can propel research on harmonization efforts in other policy contexts.

What does it all mean in practice?

Ultimately, the aim for research into drugs in sport is finding out about the human condition to enable the option of changing the world that governs the behaviour if needed. Focusing on practical implications is something that could be built into, and eventually be a characteristic strength of, a social science of drugs in sport.

A great deal has been made about the ignorance of prevalence rates. It may serve to speculate about the implications of more accurate indicators of prevalence (is it worth knowing about?). If prevalence is shown to be around 10% compared to NADO estimates of less than 2%, what does this mean in practice? An implication of this particular example is that NADOs would have to do something to bridge the gap and consequently test the resolve of those who support anti-doping. Furthering the example, the question arises as to how much extra money governments might vote towards anti-doping activity relative to other public good programmes, like vaccinations. A second apparent implication would be that while deterrence activity works on 90% of the population, it fails for 10% of the population (currently the official statistics say deterrence works for 98%). Problems emerge as to the cause of this rate, and whether such people would use irrespective of any intervention or education campaign (i.e. such campaigns are a waste of public funds).

A great deal has also been made about the system surrounding drugs in sport, such as the policy (e.g. strict liability) and stakeholder interests (e.g. interests in money rather than athlete well-being). The gap in knowledge at this juncture is to consider what effects these have on behaviour at every level (perhaps using the individual, group and organization model). There are two sets of consequences that may prove prudent to investigate: the intended and unintended, both from various perspectives. For example, the intentions of the anti-doping system may be about rescuing an Olympic-values based ideology for sport from the world of commercialized sport. The unintended consequence of anti-doping could be the creation and sustenance of the anti-doping industry, from those obviously peddling dope to those who develop public policy. Evaluating research in terms of such consequences may help make the research more useable.

One way of operationalising this potential characteristic pragmatic strength is demonstrated by Cashmore's[32] hypothetical Olympic 100m final that describes the athletes and their drug regimes. The implications that stem from this hypothetical example provide significant opportunity to explore ideas that may be unconstrained by social science dogma or fashions.[33] This form of research can be variously called war-gaming, scenario planning, future history or science fiction. Interpreting the consequences of ideas implemented with an eye to the future may lead to entirely unanticipated innovation.

The cosmopolitan research agenda

The ambitious goal of the cosmopolitan research agenda was to establish a statement to inspire collaborative research without disciplinary distinctions. The result has been a range of ideas that challenges researchers to get 'outside the square' of their own discipline and work with others to learn from each other towards innovation.

Public perception

The agenda into public perception represents a cluster of research ideas around finding out what people think about drugs in sport. The assumption that the public is opposed to drugs in sport needs to be tested. Public opinion may have evolved towards a more permissive stance that modifies the position on drugs in sport taken by the sports industry. The perception of the sports industry likewise needs to be tested. For example, has the sports industry begun to believe its own rhetoric (such as the war on drugs discourse) about drugs in sport?

Rules and effect

This area of investigation focuses on the different governing structures that are available to administer and/or police drugs in sport. This includes assessing the feasibility of different policy strategies as alternative to the anti-doping stance. The requisite corollary to policy development is the capacity to assess those policies. That is, a developed and mature set of measurements to assess policy effectiveness or achieve impartial programme evaluation must appear alongside any proposal for an alternative governing structure.

The system

Research on the system surrounding drugs in sport takes the flavour of sport management, and in particular strategic management. The first step is establishing a good understanding of the current system in terms of it strengths and weaknesses (a flag planting or benchmarking exercise). The next step is to determine where we would like drugs in sport to be (an outcome, akin to the zero tolerance policy). With the present and the future articulated to some degree, it is possible to begin mapping how to get there.

Performance enhancing behaviour

Since the late nineteenth century, sport has been a controllable microcosm of human behaviour amenable to scientific investigation, and especially performance behaviour.[34] To continue this tradition, examination of the use of PESM in relation to sport provides an opportunity to explore whether they form the basis for a set of general laws about the human pursuit of improving one's performance. For example, models developed on elite athletes may explain behaviours seen in other elite professions' pursuit of excellence (such as political, financial, legal or academic careers).

The networked athlete

There are two aspects to the research agenda associated with the networked athlete. The first is to begin researching the network surrounding the athlete. Description and analysis of the relationships that enable athletes (elite and non-elite) to participate in sport may provide invaluable insight into the unique pressures that result in prohibited PESM use. The second aspect to the networked athlete agenda is to define the lessons learned from the effort to achieve rule harmonization. This could represent an invaluable opportunity for political science and law academics to get a better understanding of how to improve the performance of international law.

In practice

All research proposed under the research agenda towards a social science of drugs in sport are subject to the caveat that they must be translated into action. At this point, the discussion is guilty of talking about talking about drugs in sport. The gravest sin that could be committed is the failure to translate this talk into action by considering the pragmatic constraints of how ideas might work in practice (researchers), or failure to listen to those who have spent significant time thinking about the ideas (practitioners). They are both sides of the same coin and need each other to have any value.

Notes

1 See Backhouse *et al.*, *Attitudes, Behaviours, Knowledge and Education – Drugs in Sport.*

2 It seems, at least to this author, that social science spends a lot of time deconstructing human behaviour into ever smaller bits, without reconciling these highly specific explanations into broader explanations of the human condition. Cosmopolitan research, as articulated here, is an expression of the idea that disciplines within social science need to reconstruct their results into explanations of the human condition that go beyond internal consistency within a given discipline or sub-discipline.

3 See Hoberman, *Mortal Engines*, 68, for a comparable explanation.

4 This anxiety is outlined by Carstairs, 'The Wide World of Doping', and to a lesser extent Lincoln Allison, 'Faster, Stronger, Higher'. *Guardian*, August 9, 2004. http://www.guardian.co.uk/g2/story/0,3604,1278957,00.html; and refuted in Miah, *Genetically Modified Athletes*, and Tamburrini, 'Are Doping Sanctions Justified? A Moral Relativistic View'.

5 See Allison, 'Faster, Stronger, Higher'.

6 This point is persuasively argued by Bette and Schimank, 'Coping with Doping: Sport Associations under Organisational Stress'.

7 This particular approach is advocated by Savulescu, Foddy and Clayton, 'Why We Should Allow Performance Enhancing Drugs in Sport'.

8 See Foster, 'The Discourses of Doping', analysis for an introduction. There also commentaries on the discourses of health risk arguments from Savulescu, Foddy and Clayton, 'Why We Should Allow Performance Enhancing Drugs in Sport', and the 'war on drugs in sport' or zero tolerance policies defined as characteristic of political discourses noted by Mendoza, 'The War on Drugs in Sport'.

9 The argument supporting the involvement of each of these is presented by Mazanov, 'Measuring Athlete Attitudes Towards Drugs in Sport'. Eiser, *Attitudes, Chaos and the Connectionist Mind*, describes how dynamical modelling of attitudes can explore how attitudes fluctuate over time and what causes that fluctuation. Finn and Louviere, 'Determining the Appropriate Response to Evidence of Public Concern', report an accessible example of best-worst scaling. In its basic form, best-worst scaling asks respondents to indicate which of several options is their most and least preferred. The options are presented several times in different combinations to model which of several options is considered to best reflect their position and which is considered to be the worst reflection. The stochastic modelling and psychometrics underlying best-worst scaling is significantly more complicated than described here.

10 See, for example, Mike Agostino, 'Drugs in Sport – Just Get Over It'. *Sydney Morning Herald*, August 5, 2006. http://www.smh.com.au/news/sport/drugs-in-sportjust-get-over-it/2006/08/04/1154198330907.html.

11 Bird and Wagner, 'Sport as a Common Property Resource'.

12 Savulescu, Foddy and Clayton, 'Why We Should Allow Performance Enhancing Drugs in Sport'.

13 For a variant of this approach in relation to cycling see E. Almond, 'Tour of California: Some Teams Take Action in Own Hands'. *Mercury News*, February 22, 2007. http://www.mercurynews.com/mld/mercurynews/sports/16762725.htm; and J. Macur, 'Welcome Testing, Team Battles Cycling's Image'. *New York Times*, February 13, 2007. http://www.nytimes.com/2007/02/13/sports/othersports/13cycle.html?pagewanted=2&_r=1&ei=5094&en=701f4b476f18fe86&hp&ex=1171342800&partner=homepage.

14 Miah, *Genetically Modified Athletes*.

15 This point came up in conversation with D. Hemphill on January 30, 2007, when discussing issues facing sport philosophy.

16 For a political scientist's efforts to reconcile this point, see Houlihan, 'The World Anti-Doping Agency: Prospects for Success'.

17 Miah, *Genetically Modified Athletes*, 36.

18 Girginov, 'Creating a Corporate Anti-doping Culture'; Houlihan, 'Anti-doping Policy in Sport'.

19 Leonard, 'Doping in Elite Swimming: A Case Study of the Modern Era from 1970 Forward', argues that the eventual anti-doping activity by FINA was driven by concerns about brand protection.

20 An official history from WADA is available at http://www.wada-ama.org/en/dynamic.ch2?pageCategory.id=312. Academic histories, in addition to the one put together for this collection (Mazanov and McDermott, The Case for a Social Science of Drugs in Sport), include Hoberman, *Mortal Engines*; Verroken, 'Drug Use and Abuse in Sport'; Voy, *Drugs, Sport, and Politics*. Popular press examples, can be found at, http://news.bbc.co.uk/sport1/hi/in_depth/2000/drugs_in_sport/859851.stm or http://observer.guardian.co.uk/osm/story/0,,1140775,00.html. A comprehensive account of the history of WADA is presented by Todd and Todd, 'Significant Events in the History of Drug Testing and the Olympic Movement: 1960–1999'. Parisotto, *Blood Sports*, describes the development of the EPO test.

21 Using economic jargon, in the sense argued by Niskanen, *Bureaucracy and Representative Government*.

22 The legitimacy of anti-doping efforts has been identified as a key issue by several authors, such as Donovan *et al.*, 'A Conceptual Framework for Achieving Performance Enhancing Drug Compliance in Sport'; Hoberman, *Mortal Engines*; and Voy, *Drugs, Sport, and Politics*.

23 Kerr, 'On the Folly of Rewarding A, While Hoping for B'.

24 Miah, *Genetically Modified Athletes*, 37.

25 Thanks to Michaela Holloway from the Australian Securities and Investment Corporation for providing a sounding board that led to this observation.

26 Such as that being conducted in Ireland by Kirby *et al.*, 'Cheating and Doping in Sport'.

27 Girginov, 'Creating a Corporate Anti-doping Culture'.

28 Thanks to Jill Owen from UNSW@ADFA for reinterpreting this idea into the language of project management.

29 This point has been explored by the British Medical Association in BMA, *Drugs in Sport: The Pressure to Perform.*

30 *OECD Environmental Strategy: 2004 Review of Progress.* http://www.oecd.org/dataoecd/51/57/31418999.pdf.

31 Houlihan, *Dying to Win*, Chapter 7.

32 As used in Allison, 'Faster, Stronger, Higher'.

33 Ways to achieve this are articulated in Root-Bernstein, *Discovering: Finding and Solving Problems at the Frontiers of Science.*

34 Hoberman, *Mortal Engines.*

References

Backhouse, S., J. McKenna, S. Robinson, and A. Atkin. *Attitudes, Behaviours, Knowledge and Education – Drugs in Sport: Past, Present and Future.* Montreal: WADA, 2007.

Bette, K.-H., and U. Schimank. 'Coping with Doping: Sport Associations under Organisational Stress'. In *Proceedings from the Workshop 'Research on Doping in Sport*, 51–69. Oslo: Research Council of Norway, May 2001.

Bird, E.J., and G.G. Wagner. 'Sport as a Common Property Resource. A Solution to the Dilemmas of Doping'. *Journal of Conflict Resolution* 41 (1997): 749–66.

BMA. *Drugs in Sport: The Pressure to Perform.* London: BMJ Publishing Group, 2002.

Carstairs, C. 'Wide World of Doping: Drug Scandals, Natural Bodies, and the Business of Sports Entertainment'. *Addiction Research and Theory* 11, no. 4 (2003): 263–81.

Donovan, R.J., G. Egger, V. Kapernick, and J. Mendoza. 'A Conceptual Framework for Achieving Performance Enhancing Drug Compliance in Sport'. *Sports Medicine* 32, no. 4 (2002): 269–84.

Eiser, J.R. *Attitudes, Chaos and the Connectionist Mind.* Oxford: Blackwell, 1994.

Finn, A., and J.L. Louviere. 'Determining the Appropriate Response to Evidence of Public Concern: The Case of Food Safety'. *Journal of Public Policy and Marketing* 11, no. 1 (1992): 12–25.

Foster, K. 'The Discourses of Doping: Law and Regulation in the Way against Drugs'. In *Drugs and Doping in Sport: Socio-Legal Perspectives*, edited by J. O'Leary, 181–203. London: Cavendish Publishing, 2001.

Girginov, V. 'Creating a Corporate Anti-doping Culture: The Role of Bulgarian Sports Governing Bodies'. *Sport in Society* 9, no. 2 (2006): 252–68.

Hoberman, J.M. *Mortal Engines: The Science of Performance and the Dehumanisation of Sport.* New York: Free Press, 1992.

Houlihan, B. 'Anti-doping Policy in Sport: The Politics of International Policy Co-ordination'. *Public Administration* 77 (1999): 311–34.
Houlihan, B. 'The World Anti-Doping Agency: Prospects for Success'. In *Drugs and Doping in Sport Socio-legal Perspectives*, edited by J. O'Leary, 125–45. London: Cavendish Publishing Limited, 2001.
Houlihan, B. *Dying to Win*. 2nd ed. Strasbourg: Council of Europe Publishing, 2.
Kerr, S. 'On the Folly of Rewarding A, While Hoping for B'. *Academy of Management* 18, no. 4 (1975): 769–83.
Kirby, K., A. Moran, S. Guerin, and T. MacIntyre. 'Cheating and Doping in Sport: An Analysis of Relevant Psychological Variables.' Paper presented at the Conference on Ethics and Social Science Research in AntiDoping, Larnaca, Cyprus, April 2006.
Leonard, J. 'Doping in Elite Swimming: A Case Study of the Modern Era from 1970 Forward'. In *Doping in Elite Sport: The Politics of Drugs in the Olympic Movement*, edited by W. Wilson and E. Derse, 225–39. Champaign, IL: Human Kinetics, 2001.
Mazanov, J. 'Measuring Athlete Attitudes towards Drugs in Sport'. In *Proceedings for the ACSPRI Social Science Methodology Conference 2006*. Sydney: ACSPRI, December 2006.
Mendoza, J. 'The War on Drugs in Sport: A Perspective from the Front-line'. *Clinical Journal of Sport Medicine* 12 (2002): 254–8.
Miah, A. *Genetically Modified Athletes: Biomedical Ethics, Gene Doping and Sport*. London: Routledge, 2004.
Niskanen, W.A. *Bureaucracy and Representative Government*. Chicago, IL: Aldine-Atherton, 1971.
Parisotto, R. *Blood Sports: The Inside Dope on Drugs in Sport*. Prahran: Hardie Grant Books, 2006.
Root-Bernstein, R.S. *Discovering: Finding and Solving Problems at the Frontiers of Science*. Cambridge, MA: Harvard University Press, 1989.
Savulescu, J., B. Foddy, and M. Clayton. 'Why We Should Allow Performance Enhancing Drugs in Sport'. *British Journal of Sports Medicine* 38 (2004): 666–70.
Tamburrini, C. 'Are Doping Sanctions Justified? A Moral Relativistic View'. *Sport in Society* 9, no. 2 (2006): 199–211.
Todd, J., and T. Todd. 'Significant Events in the History of Drug Testing and the Olympic Movement: 1960–1999'. In *Doping in Elite Sport: The Politics of Drugs in the Olympic Movement*, edited by W. Wilson and E. Derse, 65–128. Champaign, IL: Human Kinetics, 2001.
Verroken, M. 'Drug Use and Abuse in Sport'. In *Drugs in Sport*, 4th ed., edited by D.R. Mottram, 29–63, New York: Routledge, 2005.
Voy, R. *Drugs, Sport, and Politics*. Champaign, IL: Leisure Press, 1991.

Towards a social science of drugs in sport

Jason Mazanov

School of Business, UNSW@ADFA, Canberra, Australia

With the role of social science becoming more prominent in drugs in sport research, this essay sets out an agenda designed to provide a starting point for co-ordinated research in the field. The agenda is derived from efforts across the social sciences, including sports philosophy, sociology, economics, law and psychology (health and educational). These disciplinary statements are augmented by a statement on 'cosmopolitan research', aiming to establish collaboration as the norm for investigations of drugs in sport using social science methods. Some consideration is given to the practicalities of researching in this area, specifically sources of funding and working with national anti-doping organizations. This agenda and consideration for practicalities is the culmination of efforts from a team of social scientists seeking to promote research by posing questions and offering opinions with which to agree and disagree; that is, moving towards a vibrant social science of drugs in sport.

The anti-doping stance taken in the 1960s led to a very successful medical and physical science of drugs in sport. While there is much more to learn, the medical and physical sciences have developed vibrant, sophisticated models that have matured into the detection-based deterrence strategy. With that maturation comes experience in how to use detection-based tools by those seeking to promote and those seeking to undermine the anti-doping stance. Both approaches to the anti-doping stance have exposed the strengths and weaknesses of detection-based deterrence, leading the sports industry to consider alternatives. One viable alternative model that has emerged is based on the principles of prevention-based deterrence, an approach which bears the character of a social, rather than a medical or physical science. At the time of writing this agenda, there was little on the social science of drugs in sport that could inform any deterrence strategy. The development of the agenda tested whether social science could contribute to drugs in sport with an extended discussion across five social science disciplines (philosophy, law, economics, sociology and psychology). This discussion demonstrated the pressing need to create a social science of drugs in sport equal in vibrancy, sophistication and maturity to that of the medical and physical sciences.

This essay is intended to stimulate the use of social science research methods and results to explore the role of drugs in sport. Having established an agenda, attention turns to the challenge of creating the social science of drugs in sport. That is, the challenge of moving from talking about talking about research, to talking about doing and doing research. The aim of this agenda is to inspire social science researchers to discover which of the ideas comprising the agenda have merit and which need to be consigned to the dustbin of mediocrity.

A research agenda

The research agenda emerged by asking questions. These questions first came from engaging in focused discussion at the two workshops underpinning this publication. These workshops led to each contributor reflecting on how their discipline approached the issue of drugs in sport, both in terms of existing theory and results, and in terms of where work was needed to fill gaps where existing theory and results faltered. The team then went in search of questions where disciplinary boundaries became permeable and collaborative research that makes no distinction between disciplines could emerge. These questions form the basis for the research agenda.

Sports philosophy – Dennis Hemphill[1]

Sport philosophy seeks to examine the substance of arguments used to justify aspects of sport, such as anti-drug policies and practices. Examination of these arguments demonstrates that there are inconsistencies with the way anti-drug policies and practices are justified. The attempt to resolve these inconsistencies points to some gaps in knowledge that sport philosophy might usefully explore further. For example, it would be useful to reassess the notions of 'respect for persons' and drug control in light of a growing high-performance sport culture. Another example is that anti-drug policies and practices are often associated with a 'war on drugs'. Sport philosophy needs to consider whether this metaphor is appropriate for describing and justifying the campaign against drugs in sport. Finally, a critical examination of the social interests that may be served or sacrificed by the efforts to ban drugs in sport is needed.

Discussion of these sorts of ideas leads to the following research agenda for sport philosophy:

- Examination of theories of justice (e.g. distributive and procedural) for their potential to inform anti-drug policies and practices.
- Explore the ethical assumptions and implications of alternative drug control procedures to help inform public opinion and policy on performance enhancement and drug control in sport.
- Appraise the extent to which current ethical vocabularies expand or limit our understanding of sport, performance enhancement and drug control (perhaps through discourse analysis).

Sociology – James Connor[2]

In its most basic form, sociology questions the social structures that influence human behaviour, in this case, the social structures that influence athletes towards or away from using performance-enhancing drugs. Importantly, sociology sees drug use as a social activity that occurs within a web of relationships rather than an athlete acting alone. Using the critical approach common to sociology it becomes readily apparent that sport, despite its reputation, is neither fair nor particularly health enhancing. Arguably, sport is about winning, making a profit and furthering the political interests of nations. The sociologically critical approach to drugs in sport demonstrates that sociology has already done a lot of work on issues around drugs and around sport; more work could be done on creating a sociology of drugs *in* sport, however. What this suggests is that sociology could do more in communicating and disseminating the results it has already established as a framework for other social science disciplines to explore drugs in sport issues.

The ideas arising from a sociological analysis of drugs in sport proposes three key directions for future research:

- Engaging an in-depth exploration of the 'networked' athlete to get a better sense of the social circumstances that surround drug use in sport.
- Establishing whether the anti-doping stance reflects the attitudes, beliefs and/or desires of the public (e.g. does the public want drug-free sport more than they want spectacle?).
- Utilize existing, and develop novel and innovative, ways of estimating the incidence (prevalence) of performance-enhancing drug use among both elite and non-elite athletes.

Economics – Keiran Sharpe

Using the assumption that the social world is rational, economists compare models of how the world would work if it were rational (one version of reality) against what actually happens. In the context of drugs in sport, this might mean looking at what incentives exist to create a set of circumstances where the optimal rational outcome is for an athlete to use performance-enhancing drugs. Such analysis leads to a theoretical policy of how drugs in sport should be incentivised to achieve certain outcomes, and the structures required to regulate those policies. That is, economics seeks to find the rationally optimal policy that gives effect to the desired outcome; the law then seeks to find a way of designing the rules to give effect to the policy (see below). Analysis of the external regulation of anti-doping suggests alternative approaches might be preferred, such as refocusing on amateur sport to create a culture of abstinence. An alternative to external regulation is internal regulation, or regulation by the athletes for the athletes.

Underlying this analysis is the assumption that the public really wants drug-free sport, an assumption which remains to be tested using the scientific method. As such, the agenda is slanted towards testing the only policy currently in action, anti-doping. The agenda for economics looks to build an economics of drug use in sport by:

- Building a general economic theory of drug usage and drug abatement in sport. More specifically, this would require significant research into what stakeholders want, specifying utility functions for those stakeholders, and examination of how they interact.
- Once the general economic theory has been established, attention can then identify abatement strategies that can be costed relative to effectiveness (that is, cost the various abatement programmes suggested by the modelling process).
- With the economic theory in place, it becomes a matter of calibrating consequent models towards reality with empirical evidence.

Law – Anne Amos and Saul Fridman

Analysis of drugs in sport from a legal perspective looks to give effect to the existing policy (anti-doping) rather than question the effectiveness of that policy (the role of other social sciences). That is, how best to operationalise the policy using a system of rules and authority. At a crude level, the rules around anti-doping rely on strict liability (the mere presence of drugs in an athlete's system defines guilt), a range of prescribed sanctions, and a series of prescribed exemptions (such as therapeutic use exemptions [TUEs]). The authority to enforce these rules extends from the World Anti-Doping Code (WADC; as it stood in 2006) and the Court of Arbitration in Sport (CAS). The case law surrounding the implementation of this system of rules and authority revealed some gaps in knowledge from the legal perspective. Of philosophical concern was whether the policy and aims of anti-doping were being meaningfully operationalised. That is, improvements in the system of rules and authority can only be made with a greater understanding of programme effectiveness.

The agenda for the law focuses on three thematic areas for future research aimed at getting a better sense of the gap between the desired and actual effect of the current system:

- Assess the application of strict liability to drugs in sport in terms of whether it gives effect to the WADC, especially in terms of its deterrent value.
- Closer examination of the laws designed to moderate the recognized harshness of strict liability, such as grounded empirical evidence on how TUEs work in practice.
- The universality of sanctions may have varying effects on different types of athletes (e.g. a two-year ban for a gymnast *versus* a two-year ban for a golfer); research into the deterrent effect of universal sanctions across different sports may help improve the effect of the anti-doping ideology.

Health psychology – Frances Quirk

Health psychology looks at the sorts of behaviours people engage in that strengthen or diminish their health. At a general level, the contribution of health psychology to the issue of drugs has been significant. In the sports *milieu*, the work towards establishing predictors of use is somewhat limited by the absence of crucial contextual data, like prevalence of use and how vested interests might contaminate results. These pragmatic issues aside, the health psychologist's ongoing interest in models of social cognition, addiction, stress and coping, body image and personality provides a strong theoretical and empirical tradition in which to base research into drugs in sport. For example, health psychology is well practiced in looking for behaviours that show similar characteristics to those of interest and using them to effectively explore sensitive issues; in this case, performance-enhancing supplement use may be a viable substitute for performance-enhancing drug use. With a firm relationship to therapeutic (clinical) psychology, health psychology also brings data collection methods that may be missed by other social sciences, such as motivational interviewing.

The research agenda from health psychology is:

- Establishing a clear epidemiology of drugs in sport (including co-morbidity with issues like supplement use or other drug use) in the context of broad sampling frames.
- Assess whether models and theories of health behaviour can be applied in the sports context (at the elite, collegiate and amateur levels) using techniques from therapeutic practice to augment more traditional forms of research.
- Address drugs in sport as a 'systems' issue by taking into account the inter- and intra-individual differences that influence behaviour.

Educational psychology – James Hanson

The role of educational psychology, at least in terms of the constructivist approach, is to help people learn ways to make informed decisions based on a critical evaluation of their own and others beliefs, in this case, helping athletes make informed decisions about their drug use. The traditional approach to teaching via knowledge transmission has met with limited success, leading to the exploration of other forms of education (in this case constructivist approaches arising from the work on Piaget's and Vygotsky's work) to improve the retention of information, and the learner's ability to use the information available to them at the crucial moment a decision is needed. Structuring athlete education around these principles leads to clear recommendations for the design of such programmes. Elements important to educational success in this regard include interactions among learners, development of dialogic inquiry, modelling enquiry, and the principles of critical enquiry known as knowledge building.

The main thrust for the research agenda from educational psychology is determining which aspects of this model, or a model which evolves through rigorous evaluation of the current model, works best to achieve the ends of the prevailing drugs in sport policy (such as anti-doping). This means the agenda from educational psychology points to:

- A critical empirical examination of how effective existing education programmes have been; that is, programme evaluation.
- Building an understanding of how much athletes know about drugs in sport towards developing education programmes that establish 'deep' learning.
- Exploring the differential effects of education programmes over the course of athletic careers (from pre-adolescent to 'masters' athlete), including principles of adult education.

Cosmopolitan research

Where individual disciplines contribute significantly to the knowledge base, there is also scope to look for innovative synergies across social science disciplines that build towards general explanations of human behaviour. Three questions to which any social science could meaningfully contribute were used. The first question explored whether the public perceptions about drugs in sport matched those espoused by the institutions with a vested interest in sport. A starting point for approaching this problem may be a discourse analysis across the media and qualitative data collection across interest groups that feeds into a subsequent large scale quantitative survey. The second question was critical of whether the anti-doping rules were effective and called for exploration of alternatives. The third question looked at the WADA system governing drugs in sport by evaluating it closely to find out where it worked, where it could be improved, and how lessons from the WADA system could be applied to other social issues (e.g. climate change). Looking at what questions were common across different disciplines suggested work towards establishing a social science of performance-enhancing behaviour, and developing a picture of the 'networked athlete'.

A central theme that needs to run through all social science research into drugs in sport is that it must be translated into action. This means the producers of research developing work that is translatable into action, and the consumers of research translating those ideas into action (and providing feedback as part of the research effort). The direction suggested by the cosmopolitan research agenda is:

- Find out what people think about drugs in sport.
- Establish which ideology, including its governance and administration (e.g. programme evaluation), represents the most effective way to manage drugs in sport (relative to anti-doping as the null model). Such research could lead to the development of a list of 'lessons learned' from the approach to drugs in sport (ideologically and managerially) that might be applicable to other social contexts.
- Find out whether the rules governing performance-enhancement behaviour in sport can be generalized to performance enhancement in other contexts (e.g. organizational, academic or cosmetic).

A research agenda

This agenda is by no means comprehensive or complete. It reflects the ideas and issues discovered by addressing the question of how various social science disciplines could contribute to exploring and explaining the drugs in sport phenomena and was never seen as an end point. This short list of disciplines represents a departure point for the social science research effort into the drugs in sport phenomena; further contributions are necessary from disciplines such as political science, sports history, sports management, sport psychology, psychosomatic medicine and psychiatry to name a few. It is an exciting prospect to consider what these disciplines can bring to a social science of drugs in sport.

Future challenges

Creating a social science of drugs in sport means shifting the focus of social science research activity on drugs in sport: from talking about research to doing research. This raises some questions on what the future holds for creating this social science. This discussion of the future for a social science of drugs in sport is based around two key challenges that need to be approached simultaneously around conducting and disseminating research. The first simultaneous challenge is structuring the research efforts to be pragmatic. The kind of pragmatism that needs to be fostered looks to meet the needs of basic research that might be more interesting to the researcher (answering questions about the human condition) and applied research that might be more interesting for the practitioner (research that works towards resolving problems facing sport now). The second simultaneous challenge is getting the social science 'off the ground' by using the existing structures around research, such as funding opportunities.

Fostering basic and applied research

Part of the fostering of basic and applied research is ensuring that practitioners and researchers collaborate towards the common goal of understanding enough about drug use in sport to do something about it. Researchers and practitioners need to work together. Using national anti-doping organizations (NADOs) as an exemplar practitioner, collaborations with basic researchers would allow NADOs to evolve their programmes as new results from basic research come to light and define mature prevention models. Likewise, social scientists need to engage with NADOs by listening to NADOs as consumers of research. The applied research questions that interest NADOs could lead to basic research as fundamental questions become apparent. This would achieve the social scientist's goal of understanding the human condition while providing useful information that helps those with an interest in sport achieve their goals. However, the relationship between basic and applied research is sometimes difficult to find. Two examples are provided as a starting point for considering how basic and applied research co-exist in this context.

Some effort has been expended throughout this book arguing about the system surrounding drugs in sport, such as the policy (e.g. strict liability) and stakeholder interests (e.g. interests in money rather than athlete well-being). These sorts of abstract questions may have little effect on individual athletes far removed from the system, and thus of little interest to practitioners. The basic researcher might see a rich vein of research to explore how intended and unintended consequences of social systems arise. For example, the intentions of the anti-doping system may be about rescuing an Olympic-values based ideology for sport from the world of commercialized sport. The unintended consequence of anti-doping is the creation of an anti-doping industry which perpetuates commercialized sport. This basic research has significant implications for the individual athlete who can then navigate the old system more effectively or benefit from a more refined system.

The applied context can also help basic research, through, for example, efforts to calibrate the basic questions. A very pragmatic issue facing drugs in sport research is ignorance of prevalence rates. Applied research into how best to approach the measurement of prevalence could lead to some important results for basic research. For example, if prevalence is shown to be around 10% (compared to NADO estimates of less than 2%), NADOs become very interested in research that looks to understand where the 8% error came from and how to resolve the problem. This sharpens the focus of both practitioners and basic researchers to find out what principles exist to bridge the gap. Extending the example, the question arises as to how much extra money governments might vote towards anti-doping activity relative to other public good programmes, like vaccinations.

Getting social science off the ground

It has been suggested that drugs in sport research is beholden to a medical hegemony, and has been since the 1930s. If true, this means that the industry is currently skewed towards supporting medical, rather than social, research. For example, an informal survey of four organizations offering financial support for anti-doping research through their 2005 rounds showed only 10 social science or 'ethics' projects were funded compared with 129 medical science projects, with WADA the world leader in supporting social science research. This brief survey indicates that social science needs to be more innovative in getting the support needed to engage with drugs in sport research.

Given that research into drugs in sport contributes to the public good, governments are in an excellent position to address the imbalance. Some governments already have (e.g. the Australian and British Governments). However, public funds tend to be spread thinly. Social science needs to be more entrepreneurial in seeking funding, and may do well to remember that the issue of drugs in sport is highly relevant to a private sector sports industry that commands very large sums of money. Some private entities already contribute to social science based drugs in sport research, such as the IOC through WADA. Social scientists may need to be more entrepreneurial in seeking funds to support research by approaching private entities with an interest in drugs in sport research, such as:

- international sporting organizations (e.g. FIFA),
- national sporting organizations (e.g. national football leagues),
- pharmaceutical companies (e.g. producers of sports drugs),
- manufacturers of supplements (e.g. vitamin or protein supplements),
- manufacturers of sporting equipment (e.g. shoes or weights), or
- sponsors seeking to associate products with a positive sporting image.

Alternatively, governments could seek and administer funds from the sporting organizations noted above to ensure organizations with an interest in drugs in sport research are contributing to the research effort (irrespective of whether medical or social methods are used). The aim would be for the private organizations that profit from sport-related activity to benefit from research that improves the understanding of the role of drugs in sport, and public good would be enhanced as a result of governments and NADOs identifying the best way of approaching the drugs in sport issue.

However, research amounts to very little unless it is converted into something useable. Where the results from medical science are tangible and can be translated into an observable effect relatively quickly, results from social science can take longer to implement. This means that in addition to production, social science needs to be meticulous in educating consumers about research. This education comes in two ways. The first is educating those in power about the value of social science research. The second is by giving consumers the capacity to use the tools created by social science to understand the drugs in sport issue. Social science needs to move beyond saying what 'should' be done and identify ways to promote implementation as part of their research effort. The important message is that both producers and consumers of research take responsibility for making research useful.

An ambitious way of getting the social science of drugs in sport off the ground would be to pursue the establishment of an international research centre. Such a centre would promote collaborative research between the various disciplines in social science, allowing results from one discipline to inform the research of another. At its core, an international research centre would need to receive arms length funding to achieve the goal of providing objectively valid and reliable research to inform the debate about the role of drugs in sport.

Towards a social science of drugs in sport

With an agenda for a social science of drugs in sport established, the future promises to be a challenging and rewarding one. For researchers the agenda presents an opportunity to conduct innovative research on an issue of social significance. For the sports community the agenda holds the promise of significantly more scientifically derived information about drugs in sport in the public domain upon which to base decisions about policy, education or spectators deciding whether to support a team. The stated aim of this agenda was to inspire social science researchers to discover which ideas have merit and which need to be consigned to the dustbin of mediocrity. If the agenda can inspire researchers, policy makers or commentators to engage with, or pose better questions than those raised it has achieved its purpose of starting the process towards developing a social science of drugs in sport.

Notes

1 Many thanks to Dennis Hemphill for providing the notes that led to this summary.
2 Many thanks to James Connor for providing the notes that led to this summary.
3 The author acknowledges other research programs reported by non-English web sites or agencies (e.g. university grant schemes) may offer significant financial support to this line of research that would change this particular result.

Index

The Routledge Physical Education Reader

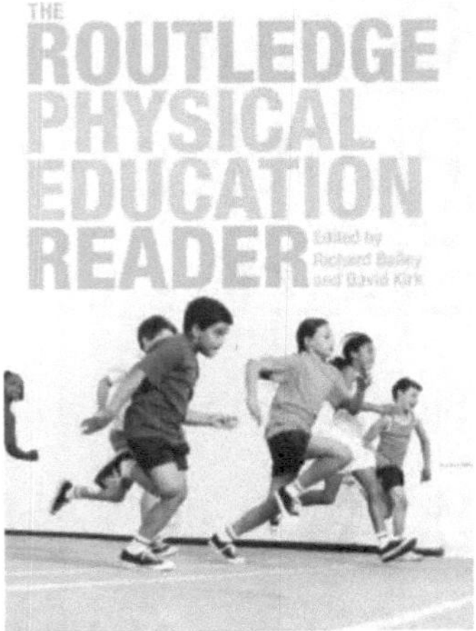

Richard Bailey
University of Birmingham UK
David Kirk,
Leeds Metropolitan University, UK

Physical Education teaching and research is fundamental to the physical and social health of our communities. The Routledge Physical Education Reader presents an authoritative and representative selection of the very best international scholarship in PE, drawn from across the full topical range of the discipline.
Containing a rich blend of contemporary, 'classic' and hard-to-find articles, this book helps students gain a full understanding of the historical context in which current issues and debates within PE have emerged. Leading international scholars Richard Bailey and David Kirk weave a thoughtful editorial commentary throughout the book that illuminates each key theme, making insightful and important connections between articles and approaches.

Contents

September 2008
PB: 978-0-415-44601-3: **£29.99** / HB: 978-0-415-44600-6: **£95.00**

Routledge
Taylor & Francis Group